IT CAN'T HAPPEN TO ME

"It was a shock to me. I thought, 'Man, Jim Irwin had a heart attack.' Someone who's as physically fit as I am. I have always been a physical fitness nut . . . I prided myself so much on being strong and healthy."

—Col. James B. Irwin, retired NASA astronaut. Two heart attacks plus bypass surgery.

"I didn't figure I'd be a man with bypasses in me. . . . In 1979, I started having these pains in my chest. One thing the doctors thought it might be was my heart. So they did an angiogram. That didn't bother me. I knew I'd be OK—I knew there'd be nothing wrong with my heart."

—Fred Rizk, president of Rizk Construction Co., Houston. Diagnosis: angina pectoris; bypass surgery recommended.

"It was a fluke. It didn't happen. All I heard was, 'How can a guy like you have a heart attack? You're the easiest going guy in the world.' That was my outward appearance, I guess, to everybody."

—Alan Keiser, retired businessman. Two heart attacks, bypass surgery, cardiac arrest, heart failure.

Also by Berkley

LIVE LONGER NOW
THE OFFICIAL PRITIKIN GUIDE TO RESTAURANT EATING

PRITIKIN PEOPLE

Penelope B. Grenoble, Ph.D.

BERKLEY BOOKS, NEW YORK

PRITIKIN PEOPLE

A Berkley Book / published by arrangement with
the author

PRINTING HISTORY
Berkley trade paperback edition/October 1986

ISBN: 0-425-09215-1

A BERKLEY BOOK® TM 757,375
Berkley Books are published by Berkley Publishing Corporation,
200 Madison Avenue, New York, NY 10016.
The name ''BERKLEY'' and the stylized ''B'' with design
are trademarks belonging to the Berkley Publishing Corporation.

PRINTED IN CANADA

Acknowledgments

Once begun, a book becomes simultaneously a fluid process and an unrelenting, static pressure. Try as you will to put it out of your mind for a day or a weekend's rest, the book is always with you—and with those around you.

And so, I owe much gratitude and thanks to my husband Phillip Myers, who spent a year of his life living with *Pritikin People*. Not only did he provide moral support but acted as copy editor, proofreader and research assistant. Without his help, this would have been grim work indeed.

To Dr. Herbert Tanney—who has guided our family through many years of ups and downs but has always managed to keep us healthy— many thanks for his careful reading of the final manuscript.

Thanks also to my agent, Jack Artenstein, for his continued support and enthusiasm for this project. And to Mary Ann Fisher, editor of *Westways* magazine in Los Angeles, for arranging time for me to work on the manuscript.

Years ago, it was customary for writers to thank their dedicated typists who foraged their way through repeated manuscript drafts. Times have changed, however, and it is with deep respect for their technical skills that I acknowledge Earl Dennis and Torsten Hoff of Computer Showcase in Los Angeles, who kept my Kaypro 10 working throughout the intense work of transcribing tapes and completing the book.

To my father,
who always answered my questions
and my mother,
who gave me vision and urged me forward.

Introduction

For two years, I worked with Nathan Pritikin as executive director of the Pritikin Research Foundation. Consulting directly with Pritikin and his advisors, I oversaw implementation of the Foundation's research projects and directed its information and education programs. The goal of our work was to document the effectiveness of the Pritikin Program in controlling degenerative disease and to raise public awareness of the role of good diet and adequate exercise as protection against illness, particularly heart disease. With more than a dozen years in the health field—as a writer, editor and filmmaker—I was intrigued by the prospect of educating people about the possibilities of disease prevention.

One of the most rewarding aspects of my job involved visiting former participants from the Pritikin Longevity Center in Santa Monica, California. Time and again I was struck by the pervasive trauma of heart disease and the quiet courage of the innumerable individuals who simply refused to be daunted by an illness that kills some 500,000 of us annually and has undermined the quality of life for millions of others.

Heart disease has an insidious "diffusion effect." From the center, or heart patient, emanate waves of shock that often upset relationships within families and between colleagues and co-workers. The after-effects of heart disease can destroy years of intimacy with one's closest friends and leave in the wake feelings of confusion, isolation, fear and desperation. In actuality, there are significant "effects" that can be felt long before an actual heart attack or *any* indication of serious illness. This is especially true of people who lead complicated, goal-ridden lives, those described as exhibiting the so-called Type A personality. People who must always live on the edge, they are the never satisfied over-achievers, absent fathers, distracted mothers, impatient bosses, good-time friends as driven about their leisure time as they are obsessed about their work. They are people for whom accomplishment is essential to self-concept and self-esteem, victims all of the ultimate American dream—That perseverance and hard work will bring reward.

Post-heart attack life, however—often the result of such driven, intense life-styles—can be devastating. For too many sufferers, heart disease means endless years of compromised living, a severely circumscribed, even zombie-like existence, in which fear and hopelessness eclipse once familiar feelings of zest, vitality, stamina and opportunity. Routinely, the heart patient's reality includes rounds of stupefying medication and/or repeated hospitalization. For them is the ever-present fear of doing too much accompanied by an equally pervasive sense of incapacity or inadequacy. The result is confusion and frustration, disorientation, anger and depression, often amplified by a profound sense of futility; Why me? Why am I still alive? As one patient put it, "Americans fear *sudden death* from a heart attack. But the reality is much worse."

I remember when I was a child, the accepted "inevitable" truth of heart disease was death. For the victim of a heart attack, life was over; people hovered around, trying tentatively to anticipate needs, but knowing always that they shouldn't expect too much—that for all intents and purposes, this person's life was over.

With each new Pritikin patient I interviewed, however, I became increasingly convinced that reality had changed. For as sure as the fact of heart disease may mean years of fear and frustration—rather than the relative relief of a swift and immediate death—the "aftermath" can be a full and productive life. And so, this book was born initially of the belief that, armed with knowledge and understanding of the realities of heart disease, we could get control of this lethal killer and might even succeed in its prevention.

At closer look, however, *prevention* seemed an insufficient objective. There remained the essential reality of those individuals who, having already experienced an attack, wrestle daily with life and the struggle to rebuild a shattered self-concept. And there are also those unfortunate others who exist daily with the pain of angina and the fear of the "final" (fatal) attack. What could I provide for these people for whom warning was essentially useless but encouragement sorely needed?

In other words, a chronicle limited to a strictly clinical description of heart disease and its effects would be incomplete and mistakenly mired in despair. The added dimension of the experiences of people committed to reversing the effects of their illness was necessary to complete the picture. On one hand, it was essential that the material provide, through the description of the negative experiences of heart patients, the incentive to avoid a way of life that can put one squarely on the road to illness. And on the other hand—and equally important—any collection of such experiences must give inspiration to those individuals already suffering from this disease so that they may learn to pick up the pieces of their broken lives.

In many aspects, the people whose words are documented in this book are not unusual; they represent conventional images of heart patients. In one fundamental characteristic, however, they are significantly different from those images, because each has remained undaunted by disease. Though they are motivated by uniquely personal factors, this common determination abides—they have refused to be maligned by their illness and have been able to summon sufficient emotional and intellectual resources to turn the tables and wrest control for themselves. How each managed to find this strength was the story I felt needed to be told.

Just how each story would unfold was a matter of close and careful deliberation. There are many approaches to organizing a collection of profiles such as this, the typical one being a rather disinterested, "objective" accounting of the medical case study, a factual approach concluded in detached, impersonal language. But having spent time with each of these individuals, and others like them, having known them over a period of years—some better than others—I rejected this methodology. Their experiences are too intimate, too personal, too full of powerful images to be reduced to mere facts and figures buried in medical reports and third-person reporting.

And so, although recognizing always the necessity of maintaining the reporter's critical eye, I opted for the role of observer-recorder, proceeding as one who questions and probes past the obvious to discover the commonality of experience in order to understand the emotions buried under neutral words and phrases. In telling their stories, I have sought the universality in the lives of these six people so that their experiences might strike a chord in others, specifically in those who now suffer from heart disease, their families and friends, as well as those others among us who fear this deadly illness and seek ways to protect ourselves against it.

So said, allow me to introduce this exemplary sextet. Each of these individuals—five men and one woman—is a master of imagination and planning, an expert at achievement. Each has a forceful personal vision, and not one among them is inclined toward compromise. These are people who are not disposed to taking orders, or waiting for others to define need and prescribe action. Could any one of these "captains" settle for a position among the crew? Not likely.

Alan Keiser is a former owner-partner in a heavy industrial supply business. His job was "to run the yards," to see that things got done, directing and managing others. Jack Rutta, retired stockbroker, now investment counselor, says he likes to implement and has no desire to remake the wheel. But what he really means is that his preference is for designing the strategies for implementation. Martin Stone's specialty is designing and developing new businesses. He could spin off three projects from the challenge of getting the proverbial boat clear of the dock. And what about astronaut James Irwin? It's difficult to think that someone who had the personal vision to accomplish a voyage to the moon would cool his heels waiting for the order to "let go the lines." Or Fred Rizk, real estate developer, the most notorious breed of independent soul? There is no way he would stand around waiting for orders. And finally there is Pam Mulhair, more driven in her own way and less capable of effecting compromise than all the men—despite her sex's reputed skills at concilliation.

These six people have little in common except heart disease and their adherence to the Pritikin Program. Their common language is of cholesterol and complex carbohydrates, of the value of nonfat dairy products and daily exercise. Each can tell you quickly how far it is from the Pritikin Longevity Center to the Santa Monica Pier or, in the other direction, to the foot of the Venice Pier. Theirs is a world of treadmills and protein substitutes. Their uniform could well be the jogging suit, and emblazoned on their consciousness are the words low fat, sugar and salt. Above all, however, I found their essential support—and solace—to be a personal determination to succeed in their new lifestyle, aided by the commitment of spouses and families. Their powerful challenge is to maintain their resolution in the face of the excesses of contemporary Western society, where eating "well" seems to be synonymous with achievement and success.

These six are Pritikin People. Although each of their lives unfolds according to a radically different script, they are linked by their determined commitment to a purpose, to a style of living that is different—at least presently—from the society in which they live. Because of this commitment, they are all happy recipients of an additional lease on life. Perhaps most significantly, their stories have never before been told. Nathan Pritikin, the founder of the Pritikin Program, wrote books that abound with optimism of the success people have experienced by adhering to his diet and exercise plan. But who are those people actually? What are they like? From Pritikin's books we know them only by their cholesterol values and exercise prescriptions. How do they see themselves? What are the challenges of maintaining their new lifestyle? How do they view the illness that laid them low? These questions and others have seemingly been lost in the debate and controversy about the efficacy of program itself.

For those unfamiliar with the Pritikin Program, I offer here a few words of introduction. Be advised, however, that this is a book about people. Those interested in more detail on coronary by-pass surgery might want to consult two books, *Bypass*, by Jonathan L. Halperin, M.D. and Richard Levine, and *Bypass—A Doctor's Recovery from Open Heart Surgery* by Joseph D. Waxberg, M.D. More detailed information on the Type A personality can be obtained from Meyer Friedman's two books, *Type A Behavior*, with Raymond Rosenman, M.D. and *Treating Type A Behavior and Your Heart*, with Diane Ulmer, R.N.

Best opportunities for further study of the Pritikin Program are available through *The Pritikin Program for Diet and Exercise* and *The Pritikin Promise*, both by Nathan Pritikin.

Briefly, the Pritikin Program for Diet and Exercise was developed by Nathan Pritikin, a non-medical professional who was trained as an engineer and spent his early years as an inventor, generating numerous patents for technical products and procedures. At the age of 42, he was diagnosed with severe heart disease. According to the conventional treatment of the time, he was told only that he should slow down, avoid exercise and watch his diet. Watch his diet he did, but differently from what his doctors had expected—or recommended.

After an exhaustive search through the available literature, Pritikin pinpointed high fat and cholesterol levels as essential elements in the heart disease equation, rightfully linking them with the dietary affluence of contemporary Western society. He sought the solution to his poor health condition in the diets of underdeveloped countries, diets based primarily on complex carbohydrates—grains and fruits and vegetables— and very little animal protein. With this information, and with the help of his wife, Ilene, he devised a dietary regimen for himself and grad- ually made his way to recovery. As he regained strength and stamina, he began a moderate walking regimen. To the simple exercise prescrip- tion he later added the increased rigor and controlled pace of a treadmill until, finally, he was able to jog.

Pritikin first reported his experiences at a general meeting of the 52nd Congress of Rehabilitation Medicine and 37th Annual Assembly

Academy of Physical Medicine and Rehabilitation in 1975 and was soon after deluged with requests for help from people suffering from similar illness and its often attendant feelings of helplessness. His response was to found the Longevity Research Institute in 1977, based originally in Santa Barbara, California. The demand for his program became so great, however, that he moved to Santa Monica soon after, where he established the Pritikin Longevity Center and renamed the Longevity Research Institute the Pritikin Research Foundation, his non-profit institute dedicated to research in degenerative disease.

The core of the Pritikin Program is a diet low in fat, cholesterol, salt and sugar. Specifically this means restricting animal protein consumption—chosen from fish, chicken and turkey (preferably fresh)—to three-and-one-half ounces per day. No red meat or organ meat is allowed. All fats and oils are to be avoided on food or in cooking. Meats are sauteed in defatted chicken stock instead of oil; mashed bananas replace butter and jam on morning toast; salad dressings have a vegetable juice or nonfat yogurt base. Sugar, in all its forms, is prohibited from the Pritikin diet; in baking, fruit juices and fruit pulp are substituted for the traditional sugar, molasses or honey. Coffee, tea, chocolate and other caffeine-containing food and drink are also not allowed, and the program discourages the use of alcohol.

What can one eat may well be a justified question. To start with, large amounts of salads and freshly cooked green vegetables, along with potatoes, yams, corn, whole grains, cereals and bread, are allowed and encouraged. Reasonable servings of fruit, nonfat dairy products and lean meat—again, fresh fish, chicken or turkey—form the basis of the Pritikin Program. This is what is referred to as the Maintenance Diet, recommended for most people suffering from heart disease who have reduced their cholesterol to a suitable level (roughly between 160 and 180, depending on their health history) and those seeking to avoid such illness. For individuals suffering from excessive levels of serum cholesterol (measured by the amount of cholesterol in the blood) there is the Regression Diet, an essentially vegetarian regimen that limits animal protein to one-and-a-half ounces *a week* and reduces the amount of fruit consumed.

Regular, routine exercise is essential to the program because it increases physical stamina and strengthens the heart. Regular exercise can help lower blood pressure and lower the heart rate, and evidence suggests that exercise may also help lower blood cholesterol and alter the way existing cholesterol is carried in the blood stream. With exercise, post-heart attack victims may also develop collateral blood vessels to help nourish their damaged heart muscle. Participants at the Pritikin

Centers undergo a stress test from which a carefully prepared "exercise prescription" is recommended. Some patients opt for regular use of a treadmill, while other prefer vigorous walking. Patients with a history of heart disease are encouraged to build their stamina gradually, eventually progressing to a regular program of walking or jogging. Once settled into a regular personal routine at home, they may opt for swimming or sports such as tennis and special interest exercise such as hiking or even dancing.

In studies conducted through the research foundation and at the various centers, Pritikin and his staff have reported a number of studies based on the successful application of the Pritikin dietary and exercise program. Statistics, however, are inadequate to tell the story. As one of the individuals interviewed in this book explains, "The diet aspect of the program is simple; it's the behavior that's difficult." Which is why the experiences of these six people are so valuable. Their struggles, challenges and successes provide hope, inspiration—and insight—for you or anyone you may know who now suffers from or fears heart disease.

Chapter 1

Alan Keiser, 62, retired businessman. Married, four grown children.

Two heart attacks, bypass surgery, cardiac arrest, heart failure.

Diagnosis: severe heart disease.

I

"It was a fluke; it didn't happen."

A stylishly dressed, youthful couple struggles to find their seats in the first-class section of a wide-bodied airplane. They are on their way from Los Angeles to Philadelphia. The stewardess helps them get settled. It's late winter, 1972, and Bea and Alan Keiser are returning from an extended business trip combined with a lengthy visit with friends in California. They have been away longer than expected—four weeks, instead of five days—and are glad to be going home. Alan is a partner in a prosperous family business and is anxious to get back on the job. Bea has left their four children in the care of a housekeeper. She is looking forward to seeing them after this unexpected long absence.

Bea and Alan make themselves comfortable in their seats. The plane takes off uneventfully and a smooth flight is forecast. A flight attendant takes the Keisers' drink order and returns with cocktails and peanuts. Husband and wife exchange small talk about their growing children and their numerous household pets, along with the things they "have to do" when they arrive home. The plane levels off at cruising altitude and the clutch of flight attendants disappears, busy with preparations for the in-flight meal. Suddenly, Alan's normally ruddy complexion fades to ghostly white. He is ominously silent. Bea quickly puts aside her drink and focuses on her husband. She is conscious that he is breathing rapidly, and with a great deal of effort.

1

Before she can speak, Alan manages a faint whisper, "I can't . . . I can't breathe," he says. And then the fearful words, "I'm having a heart attack."

Bea's response is immediate. "Where are your pills?" she asks.

"In my pocket," Alan manages.

"Can you reach them?" she questions him.

"No," he answers weakly. Bea stretches across her own seat, finds the nitroglycerin in the small vial in Alan's pants pocket and puts one under her husband's tongue. The rest is confusion.

HEART ATTACK. The words immobilize. Perhaps because the effect is immediate. Breathing is truncated, and there is pain, constriction, pressure. The victim may become unconscious, or remain awake and aware of his struggle—in which case, add anxiety to the list. Regardless, the problem demands instant attention; it will not wait for calm admission to a hospital and days, perhaps weeks, of treatment. It is impatient with proper diagnosis and treatment from white-coated medical professionals. It prefers the ministrations of paramedics and firemen, ambulance attendants and emergency-room personnel. Remedial action must be swift and specific. There is no time to lose. Time, in fact, is the enemy of the heart attack victim. Time is critical. Keep the heart going, try to minimize damage, stabilize function. And all of this is amplified by the reputation that proceeds it.

Heart attacks mean death—perhaps sooner than later—or at the very least a dramatic loss of quality of life. Even as the struggle ensues, there comes to the victim the visualization of miserable days ahead. Death, the ultimate visitor, is sometimes easier to comprehend than a life devoured by fear of another attack, the spectre of lingering death. Heart attack: the one "accident," the one emergency that supersedes all others.

Alan Keiser's experience is classic—a Hollywood script of the heart attack story. The worst scenario of a nasty disease, the ultimate, heavyweight bout with the demon in all its manifestations. First, the isolated event, soon forgotten, then another attack, then another. There is a profound sense of futility, hopelessness. Death is seemingly sitting in the next chair, riding on the shoulder. Death, a welcome friend. For Alan, the final verdict was "Take him home, there's nothing more we can do for him. Take him home, there's nothing you can do—because he has no time." Time is the enemy of the heart attack victim.

But wait, a fragile sliver of hope. Shall we take it? No, death is too close. Death is a whisper away. Death is my friend. "I knew," says Bea Keiser, "if I didn't do something, he would die. He was dying in front of me; I could see it. I just prayed that he'd stay alive long enough. I prayed that God was keeping him alive for a reason.''

The first time I heard the Keisers' story, I was overwhelmed by its enormity, and not just in terms of Alan's considerable physical suffering. This is not a one-man show. The stage is packed with a memorable supporting cast—wife, children, well-intentioned doctors, friends, in-laws, more doctors—some impatient, others frustrated. Alan was a young man—41—when he had his first heart attack, and his illness became a cloud of fear and confusion that defused itself throughout his young family. Four active children joined the script. A young wife who filled the domestic gaps created by her intense and driven mate. Bea— the woman who kept Alan alive. The woman whose spirit fought off the demon death, defied the fiend incapacity, dispelled the spectre of defeat. Without Bea, Alan Keiser would probably be dead today. And although the flag is not raised around these words, no one who is privy to the Keisers' story would dispute them. Without Bea, the children might well have become emotional cripples, contaminated by an illness that was part of their life for virtually as long as they can remember. Without her determination, her persistence, without her reverence for life, Bea herself might well have not survived these events without making companions of bitterness and despair.

Alan and Bea and their family inspired this book. My hope is that more people will come to understand the consequences of our mindless flirtation with this demanding illness—the indiscriminate selfishness of heart disease. Most of all, I hope for the understanding that it can be beaten.

HEART ATTACK—the toll, the price, the odds.

Today Alan Keiser is a man whose heart steadily refuses to function, except for the very precious fifteen percent of this vital muscle that remains living, beating. But crippled? Hardly. Robust, handsome, thin and physically fit, Alan looks like a man who has not seen a day of serious illness in his entire life. He has retired now from the family business and is active in the community. He serves on the board of a local bank and is continually involved with a long list of projects. He is a man who still walks miles each day and plays golf regularly with his wife. A man who laughs and enjoys life. A man who should have been dead and buried years ago, but who is still here and having a good go at it.

Alan's transcontinental heart attack happened thirteen years ago. Today he and Bea sit in the den of their warm and stylish Palm Beach home, remembering the events of that fateful day. Bea Keiser is eight years younger than her husband. A petite, compact woman, she looks much younger than her age. Dressed in shorts and a tank top, she moves around her house with purpose and grace. Not jumpy, but determined. There is always intent and focus to her actions—fixing lunch, searching for a book, recalling experiences, explaining the significance of an event. Alan, on the other hand, floats. While Bea steps resolutely forward, Alan eases, slides, invites less commitment. Sitting in his chair doing his needlepoint, he is the picture of an eccentric English earl, taught his precocious skill at the hands of some equally eccentric grandmother or nanny. "But," says Bea, "he wasn't always like that."

Bea is sitting across the sofa from me in what is the family room of their Palm Beach home. The gaming table she sits adjacent to is oval and at a level that can double as a dining room table. Alan has settled himself in a chair at the end of the sofa—his chair. From there he can command the room, check the patio outside and watch television. The den of the Keiser home connects directly to the kitchen. The living room runs along the front of the house and looks out on the circular driveway that welcomes you as enter from the street. An earth-colored, Mexican-style tile floor curves from the room we're in through the kitchen and into the living room. It's a very comfortable house, deco- rated in warm colors and blue, a melding of Eastern establishment conservative with Palm Beach informality—accomplished with an un- selfconscious sense of style, not overly showy or ostentatious. Off in another part of the house, the Keisers' 28-year-old son, Billy, is watch- ing the basketball game. Two dogs tumble about under our feet—a gregarious Pekinese and a timid German shepherd.

"One of the reasons he started the needlepoint," she explains, "was because it helped him to calm down. I think it's a form of some sort of meditation."

Alan agrees. "I'm sitting here talking to you, relaxed. I watch TV the same way—keeps me from nibbling so much."

"It's a wonderful way of not eating," says Bea. "We sort of figured that out. It keeps the hands going, but not going to the mouth."

We are recalling the events that followed Alan's heart attack on the airplane. Bea says she remembers reaching over and getting Alan's nitroglycerin pills out of his pocket.

I ask her how she felt when the heart attack happened on the plane.

Before Bea can answer, Alan pipes up, crowing like a rooster in praise of his wife. "Are you kidding? She took charge, period."

Bea's view is different. "It was scary," she says. "It was really, absolutely scary."

But Alan isn't finished. He says, "I never saw anybody act like she did—boom, boom boom.'' Then he adds, almost as an afterthought, ''I knew what was happening—the heart attack. I was conscious and everything. I took the nitro and I was holding my own. They were in a little bottle,'' he explains. ''They're still here, right here.'' He pats the pocket of his lightweight trousers. ''Same place. It's the only time I've ever used them.''

Bea remembers, ''I told the stewardess that I needed a doctor immediately, that Alan was having a heart attack. I asked her if there was a doctor on board, and then I told her, 'I want oxygen.' She said, 'I'll see' and went up front to push the button so the automatic oxygen would come down.'' Bea pauses. Alan smiles and says, ''It didn't work.''

''Right,'' says Bea. ''When the stewardess came back to tell me, I was incredulous. I told her there had to be some oxygen on board, that the captain must have some extra oxygen. So she went back to check and came back with a small bottle and gave it to Alan.''

''Hooked it up,'' Alan explains, ''with one of the masks.''

Bea Keiser is recounting their story very deliberately, with reflection, reaching to recall details correctly. Alan is following her recitation carefully and offering lively interjections as the account progresses. It's a recurrent pattern that seems to distinguish their conversation. He appears content to allow Bea to narrate until the account—by his standards—becomes too heavy or emotion-laden. Then he brightens and either sets the conversation on another track or attempts to inject humor or a change of pace. He listens carefully to his wife's words, beaming at her efforts on his behalf. It's obvious that he's extremely proud of her.

''And the next thing I remember saying—'' says Bea.

''About the landing,'' Alan interrupts. ''I remember every bit of it.''

''Yes,'' continues Bea. ''Then I told her, the stewardess, 'I would like the captain to come back.' The conversation went like this:

'' 'Well, the captain can't come back because he's flying the plane,' the stewardess said to me.

''To which I responded, 'Don't tell me that; it's on automatic pilot, I want him now.' So she went away and the next thing I know the captain trotted back. 'What's the matter, little lady?' he asked me.

'' 'Well, first of all,' I started, 'my husband's having a heart attack. You don't have a doctor on board and I want to know where we are and how soon can we land this plane.'

'' 'I don't know where we are exactly,' the captain said to me. But then he thought for a minute and said, 'Just a minute, I'll find out.'

"Next he came back with the flight engineer, who said that we're twenty minutes outside of Denver and forty minutes outside of Omaha. So I asked him how fast we could get the plane down.

" 'Oh,' the captain told me, 'this is a nonstop flight.'

" 'No, it's not,' I corrected him. 'We're going to put this plane down as soon as we possibly can because my husband must get to a hospital. There's no doctor on board; we're going to run out of oxygen and I want him taken care of.' "

Alan watches his wife intently as she recites the story and he continues to beam his approval of her chutzpah. Bea's voice is very even as she speaks. In fact, her expression seems to always have this smooth quality, caressing events, emotions and decisions with equal amounts of attention to word choice and editorial comment. She closes the final consonants of each word, a habit that, along with the studied pace of her speech, can make her expression seem formal. In truth, she is the least formal of people.

Moving quickly into the story now, she says, "They admitted they didn't know what we should do. So I told them, 'Well, you'll just find out where we should land.'

"So they went to the cockpit and came back and said, 'We're turning the plane over to you. Shall we go into Denver?' I remember them saying this to me. 'Or do you want to go to Omaha?' I asked them about the weather.

" 'Well,' said the captain, 'the weather in Denver is bad and we'll have to jettison fuel and drop in quickly.' As he said that, I thought to myself, 'Denver—the mile-high city; there might be a problem there with Alan. He needs oxygen; maybe it won't be such a good idea.' I knew Omaha was somewhere in the middle of the country, exactly where I wasn't sure, but the weather was good in Omaha. I also thought about what would happen to the other passengers if the plane were to crash trying to land in Denver. These were my thoughts: 'I'll have to be responsible not only for Alan but all the other people that may have a problem.' Quickly I went through this; I mean in a second this happened, and I said to them, 'We'll go to Omaha.' " She stops for a moment. "I suddenly became struck with power," she laughs as she recalls her words, "and, I told them, 'I want you to radio ahead—' "

Alan pipes in, "I heard every word of it. I can vouch for it."

Bea continues, "I told the pilot, 'This is the number of the doctor in Philadelphia, Dr. Likoff. I want him to be notified. I also want the head of cardiology at the hospital—find out exactly what hospital we're going to and it better be a good one—and I want the head of cardiology to meet us and I want him to have been in touch with our cardiologist in

Philadelphia. Because this is the only way we'll get expert service, and this is exactly what we need at this point to make sure that my husband gets better.'

"The pilot said to me, 'Well, OK, anything else?' And I'm thinking, 'Well, I wonder if we ought to call the kids,' but I decided that was enough.''

Alan chuckles in his chair. His speech is more mercurial than his wife's, tending to rise in volume and pitch when he's excited or joking, and then to soften and lower as he attacks more serious subjects. Listening to Bea tell this part of the story, his interjections are light and sharp.

Bea presses forward, taking yellow yarn and knitting needles from the basket at her feet. "So they did what I asked and we landed at the end of the runway in Omaha. Some firemen came up the ramp and onto the plane and said, 'All right, now who's the problem?' They saw Alan and then they said, 'OK, just walk to the end here.' I looked at them and said, 'What?' ''

Alan imitates the firemen, " 'Walk down the steps and we'll get you down at the bottom.' ''

"But," says Bea, "I told them he was not walking."

Alan adds, "I was getting up—always the nice guy."

"Finally," says Bea, "and I don't know why I did this, but I took Alan's shoes off and I loosened his belt so he had no pressure. And I made sure his tie was loose. Then I said to the firemen, 'Now, you're going to make one of these hand seats and you're going to carry him down the stairs and then you're going to put him on a stretcher. He's not walking.' ''

"They said to me, 'Oh, OK.' '' She pauses and says, "Although I was very quiet about it, I just can't believe that what I asked for was exactly what was done.'' Alan smiles.

"I remember after they got Alan out of the plane and into the ambulance, I stepped out so I'd remember just exactly where Omaha was. Then the pilot stepped out of the plane and down the ramp. He came over to me and grabbed my hand and said, 'Look, little lady, I'm going to tell you something: He's going to make it. If you got me'—and he pointed over at the plane—'to come from there to here, he wouldn't dare die.' Then he said it again, 'He wouldn't dare die.' These words stuck in my mind as I went into that hospital. I didn't know a soul in the world there—in the hospital or in Omaha. It was really a very scary thing.''

According to the American Heart Association, the first hours after a heart attack are critical. Of the approximate one and a half million people a year who will experience a heart attack, 350,000 of them will die before they reach the hospital. The average victim waits three hours before deciding to seek help. The Heart Association encourages anyone who is with a person who may be having an attack to get the patient help immediately and ignore the usual protestations of denial. When you realize that most people who succumb to heart attacks do so in the first two hours after the initial symptoms, you understand Bea Keiser's concern about waiting until they landed in Philadelphia to get Alan medical help. If at first her actions appear melodramatic, remember that she was well-informed about heart disease and she courageously implemented the best course of action to save Alan's life. She admits, however, that throughout the time on the plane and the period en route to the hospital, she was fearful that her husband might die.

"I was sure," she says, "that he wasn't going to make it. The doctor told me in the emergency room that his chances of surviving were none. When I called his brother and sister-in-law to come out, I told them I didn't know whether they would see him alive."

Alan breaks in and initiates the first of his subject-modifying strategies. "Yeah, I fooled them all," he chuckles. Asked how he knew he was having a heart attack, he replies, "Chest pains and the whole thing. I knew right away. But I don't think I had time to be scared. I was awake the whole time, although I have no recollection about what I was thinking. I haven't even thought about it. And," he says, as if this were the primary factor, "I knew exactly what she was doing."

Bea interrupts, "I think what it was—what Alan feels—"

But her husband stops her. "She's a take-charge person," he explains forcefully. "Sure, she'll do it. Are you kidding?"

Bea clarifies their combined thought. "Alan feels it's not his problem; it's not his problem."

Alan refuses further comment, however, and deftly changes the subject and the mood by observing, "That was a great hospital. It really was. The people in Omaha were so nice to her. Never in your life should you meet people so nice."

Bea recalls she was particularly impressed by the intensive-care unit available to heart patients in the Omaha hospital. "I was amazed at that," she says. "I remember there were five beds with a nurse sitting at the desk and everybody was hooked up to monitors. She was able to monitor everyone from her desk. That seemed to me to be pretty terrific—a major breakthrough compared to the old oxygen tent Alan had been in the first time. It was like coming out of the dark ages of cardiac care. And the people were wonderful, absolutely wonderful," she continues. "I didn't know a soul. I myself was recuperating from having a lump removed from my lung."

"This one," remarks Alan, pointing at his wife, "went through ten times more hell than I've ever gone through with hospitals and all that stuff." Then he adds, "I should have to sit with her all the time."

When I look puzzled, Bea goes on to explain. "It wasn't cancer," she says. "It was just a tumor and they took it out. I had stopped smoking, I guess about a year and a half before. Then I went in for a routine chest X ray because I was going to have a spinal fusion in my neck. I had been hit by a golf ball and it caused a whiplash. As a result, I had a pinched nerve that was giving me terrible headaches and I was losing the use of my right eye because of it. They were afraid that the disks would eventually crush and cause all kinds of problems. So getting ready to have this surgery, they did the simple chest X ray. And they said, 'Forget the neck.' This all happened in California, the surgery and all, which is why we were so late starting home to Philadelphia. One of our friends in California was a surgeon, and he wanted to clear up once and for all the problem with my neck.

"So they did the lung surgery. But," she continues, putting her knitting down on the table next to her, "they knew eventually they would have to do the spinal fusion. The doctor had told me he wanted me to do some simple exercises and also to have therapy and then eventually I would have the surgery done. I'm telling you all of this because when Al was in the hospital in Omaha, I didn't know a soul. The neighborhood wasn't the greatest and I didn't have a place to stay. So I said to the doctor, 'Do me a favor; check me into the hospital as your patient and put me in a room and let me get my back therapy. Then I'll be there—because I don't know where to go. I don't know what to do.' So they admitted me," she concludes amiably, "and if I wanted to go out, all I did was get a pass and I could go out."

Alan chortles, "We had a great setup."

In the emergency room and after, as she waited for the doctors to stabilize Alan's condition—haunted by their assessment that he wouldn't survive—Bea Keiser describes herself as "being in a holding pattern." She says, "There was very little I could do, except hope and pray that our worst fears would not be realized. I tried to keep my children calm via the telephone, and not let them know it was as bad as it was. They were sixteen—"

"Down to twelve," finishes Alan, pulling a thread deftly through his needlepoint grid.

"It was getting through those first few hours," Bea sighs. "I think I was in such a low, low point; it was like me against the world. There I was in a strange town and I didn't know anyone and yet the kindness that I saw exhibited around me helped bolster me up."

"The Midwest," chirps Alan, "is so much different from the East Coast. The people are so much nicer."

Bea agrees, "From the nurses, the doctor, to the people surrounding us—they just sort of like, cuddled us. I didn't really feel like I was horribly alone because of the people." She smiles and picks up her knitting again.

"I had the most beautiful room in that hotel," Alan says. He stops. "I mean in that hospital." He laughs briefly at his gaff and continues. "The waiting room, which was right across from my room, was a little tiny thing, so people thought my room was the waiting room. They'd walk right in. But they were all so nice, I'd sit and talk with them. They'd want to know how I was doing and everything."

Bea remembers other support from strangers. "Our son, Billy," she explains, "had a friend whose parents knew someone who lived in Omaha and these people came and adopted us. They were the sweetest, dearest people."

"They took care of Bea," remembers Alan. "They took her out to dinner, and they would bring me back little goodies like corned beef sandwiches and things." He grins and adds gleefully, "See, I still wasn't on the right food."

For the next four weeks, as his wife monitored his progress, Alan Keiser gradually but steadily recuperated from his heart attack, while Bea began preparations to take him home to Philadelphia. "I think my greatest fear," she says softly, "was having to leave Omaha, having to leave that cocoon of safety. I think I may have been in a semi-shock in the beginning. Then I was so happy to watch Alan's progress that I never thought past getting through each day. My thoughts did not go further than that. And I know there was panic within me to realize that I had to take Al on the airplane and go home. That was a *very* difficult time for me and I—"

Again Alan breaks the mood. "Nothing to it," he says. Bea responds in kind, "I know, I know, but I was very upset about that. It was very difficult for me, although I've never expressed it." Alan understands what she means, however. "Going back to that same old stuff again," he says.

But home they went, back to the life that Bea feared—fears, incidentally that were well-founded. The incident on the airplane that she had so deftly handled was Alan Keiser's second heart attack. Eight years before, when he was just over forty, an up-and-coming businessman with a growing family and a hectic life-style, he first became aware of his heart problems. Bea remembers that the family physician—an internist—refused to believe this was happening to Alan.

"The doctor was the same age as Alan and he couldn't believe that anyone that young could have a heart attack," she discloses. "I called him and told him that Alan was having pains and I thought he was having a heart attack. The doctor replied that he 'couldn't be.' He told me he was going sailing, but I insisted he come over. So on his way to go put his boat in the water, he took the time to stop by our house. He told me that Alan's problem was probably indigestion and he should take some pills for that. I maintained that I thought it was a heart attack. So he finally gave me some nitroglycerin." (Nitroglycerin has been used for patients with suspected heart disease since the last century. It helps by dilating blood vessels in various parts of the body, thus lessening the workload on the heart's pumping action.)

Since his doctor didn't suggest Alan enter the hospital, during the next twenty-four hours the Keisers attempted to go through the motions of business-as-usual. Bea concedes, "Because I let the doctor know how concerned I was, he finally said we'd see how Alan got through the night. The next morning, Alan reported, 'I'll be fine, I'll be fine, no problem.' She repeats it again, as if in testimony to the irony of the situation. 'No problem.' " Alan himself recalls having breakfast that morning and going to work and, in the evening, having company for dinner. They ate steak," he says. "A steak in those days, prepared on the grill, was considered a non-fattening meal."

With a click of her knitting needles, Bea acknowledges that she was angry at both the doctor and at Alan. "It was complete denial," she says, "super denial." And then as if to illustrate her point, she explains, "That night, Alan started to have problems. I wanted to call the doctor, but Alan insisted it couldn't be anything but a little indigestion—and that there was 'no problem.' I wasn't happy and Alan didn't really sleep that well. So we went to the doctor the next day. He did a cardiogram and said, 'I think we'll put Alan in the hospital.' "

Alan laughs meaningfully. "Yeah, mildly enough, let's get him over to the hospital, quick."

Bea goes on, "That was in 1964, and they put him in that old-fashioned oxygen tent." Remembering Omaha, she says, "You have no idea the revolutionary way that patients are treated, comparing 1964 with the way things have changed. This awful tent and we were in a horrible neighborhood. I remember the whole thing. This place was in the middle of the riots they were having in Philadelphia, the wars."

She pauses again and then says, "But Alan survived in spite of the doctor. Thank God he was in good physical shape because that attack resulted in complete closure of one artery. Fortunately they diagnosed that he had only mild coronary artery disease, not advanced, and he was able to recover well.'' She notes, however, that their doctor didn't call in a cardiologist. ''He handled it himself,'' she says, ''and we didn't know any better.''

Although their own physician seemed happy with Alan's condition, the Keisers knew of a nationally known cardiologist, who at one time was president of the American College of Cardiologists. Bea decided to set up an appointment and take Alan to see Dr. William Likoff, now retired, who had once served as director of the Cardiovascular Institute at Hahnemann Medical College and Hospital in Philadelphia. Alan says he doesn't remember how he felt during that time, except that he was weak, and—typical of Alan—that he didn't like the hospital or the food.

It's Bea's opinion that Alan was not very concerned about this initial heart attack. ''He never really thought that anything was going to happen to him,'' she says. ''He was so sure that he was going to get better and everything was going to be fine. He'd never been sick before.'' In contrast, Bea herself was very cognizant of the ramifications of Alan's illness. ''I felt like my world was going to literally collapse,'' she remembers. ''It was a terrible feeling of aloneness for me, a terrible feeling. And I think maybe it was related to the fact of the doctor's attitude—he literally couldn't understand how Alan could have had a heart attack. He kept saying things like 'It doesn't happen to people this young.' It was like he considered the whole thing a fluke. And that was sort of the attitude Alan had.''

Alan confirms her statement. ''Yes,'' he says, ''it didn't happen.''

''At first, I know,'' she says, ''my fear was that Alan might die. When he survived the initial seventy-two hours, however, I knew he was going to be all right. I had heard the first seventy-two hours were critical and after that it was up to the patient to start to handle his life and take charge of it again. So I did not feel that he was about to die. And yet,'' she grants, ''that can happen.

''Then after Alan came out of the hospital and was recuperating,'' she continues, ''I had a miscarriage and went into the hospital. While I was there, I stayed and had my tubes tied. After experiencing a number of miscarriages and having a husband that might have problems, I didn't think it was fair to the four children we had. We were at a point of making decisions about where life was going to take us. I knew I did not want to have the emotional trauma of another miscarriage—and I wanted to be able to be strong for Alan if he needed me.

''The minute I got through my little episode and I came home,'' she goes on, ''I knew that I didn't like the direction we'd been given for

Alan's recuperation and for what he should do now that he'd had a heart attack. That's why I got him to a cardiologist. I was trying to do it in a nice gentle way, so I wouldn't upset Alan and I wouldn't upset our doctor. But I wanted to get Alan on the right road. Dr. Likoff put him in the hospital for evaluation. Alan had his initial attack in July, 1964, and it was almost a year later that I finally was able gradually to set all of this up.''

Alan thinks back, "They had just started the cardiac catheterization. It was almost experimental and I can remember when I lay there on the table, there must have been a hundred doctors who were there to watch it to see what it looked like." He stops, thinks a moment further. "Even that didn't bother me." Bea adds details to his brief account of the angiogram. "Dr. Likoff had had a heart attack shortly before and he had the catheterization. So I said to Alan, 'Now if he can have the catheterization, there's no reason why you shouldn't.' ''

Although the risks associated with angiograms have been reduced as the technique has been perfected, there can be complications, primarily damage to the blood vessels caused by the catheter or the possibility that the movement of the catheter through the arteries could cause a coronary spasm or dislodge pieces of plaque or a blood clot and thus trigger a heart attack.

By the time Bea arranged for the visit to the cardiologist and for the angiogram, Alan Keiser was vigorously back at work; in fact, Alan remembers that he was back on the job a brief twelve weeks after the heart attack. Says Bea, "Alan went back a little more energetically than he should have. Although his hours were a little modified—''

"Yeah, instead of sixteen hours a day," grins Alan, putting aside his needlepoint, "it was only nine or ten."

"Before Alan's heart attack," Bea says, "he would leave at five-thirty and he'd come home at seven—''

"Eight," beams Alan, as if he's proud.

"After the heart attack," Bea continues, "he would have breakfast at home with the children and he would go into work about seven or seven-thirty in the morning and come home between six and six-thirty at night."

"In time to have dinner with the family," says her husband lightly. "Until that time, I was almost an absentee father." He hesitates and then adds, "One of the good things that came out of the whole thing was that I got to know my family because of the heart attack."

At the time of his first attack, Alan Keiser and his brother were partners in a pipe-fitting and supply business located in Philadelphia.

They had started the business with money saved from World War II bonds, so by 1964, having invested not only money but also commitment to success, the two were beginning to experience considerable fruits from their labor. Alan's job was in operations. He remembers, "We had a tremendous function in the yards. That was my part—the outside operations. It was a high-pressure business because it was competitive, but if you knew what you were doing, you could make a buck. If you knew what you were doing, and you did it big, you could make a real buck out of it. So that was our style—to give service, whether it cost you here or not." He brings his right hand to the middle of his chest near his heart, in the classic heart patient salute. "I was working at that pace for years."

Bea adds, "That's his style. He's a Type A."

"Type A modified now," says her husband, continuing with his needlepoint.

Bea, as usual, clarifies the fine points. "Alan had a different style from his brother," she explains. "His brother worked at a more normal pace while Alan was doing a hop, skip and jump. It took Alan a while to learn how to deal well with this."

"No," says Alan, "it's my nature. You do a job and you've got to do it right, period."

"He's a perfectionist, a Type A. And it was taking a toll."

"But," says Alan amiably, "I loved it. Are you kidding? It was the greatest fun I ever had in my life. When work's not fun, you leave."

Bea interrupts. "Except," she starts, "and we've never had this discussion before—psychologically sometimes—"

But Alan is still working on the first idea. "If it's stimulating, if it's something new every day, something to look forward to . . ."

Bea is not about to let her own idea drop, however. Addressing her husband, she says, "You say when it's not fun you want to get out. It's an interesting thought—not that you brought about the heart attacks yourself, but maybe it wasn't fun anymore and you were looking for a way to get out." Alan is silent for a moment, shifting in his chair, but he offers no comment on Bea's suggestion.

'As they talk, the Keisers paint a picture not dissimilar from many American families—the husband works conscientiously to fulfill his role as the breadwinner while the wife puts equal energy into raising the family. The husband-father spends long hours away from home and is disconnected from the affairs of the household, which fall almost exclusively to the wife. Spurred by a mutual desire to get ahead, it can often be a difficult pattern to break. When I asked Alan if he had any sense of missing time with his family, he answered without much thought, "Never bothered me."

Bea says life during those years was frustrating. "We never argued," she says, "because Alan was never home."

Alan fires off a round of his own. "That's all I heard from her, all the time—no time with the family. We went on family vacations and stuff."

"Not until after you had your heart attack."

"Before that we'd leave the kids home. It was a pleasure to be away, and I wanted to be with Bea. I didn't see enough of her."

Bea stops the exchange. "Then after the first heart attack, Alan stopped going in on Saturdays, or else he'd take the children with him and Saturdays became—"

"Saturdays became kids' day with me," Alan explains pleasantly. "Our plant was near the waterfront and I'd take them to see all the boats. We'd go in the plant and they'd play with machines, and I'd spend an hour or two in the office doing my work when there was nobody around. Then we'd go down to the Navy yard and watch the boats or we'd stop and watch a freighter be unloaded and we'd have lunch together. It was great."

So there were some changes in the Keiser life-style as a result of Alan's first attack, but major modifications in eating habits and exercise were not among them. "We ate the typical American diet," says Bea. "That was the beginning of the barbecuing and the greatest thing would be to grill steaks outside."

"Like every night of the week," winks Alan.

"Not every night," she corrects him. "Chicken maybe once or twice a week, occasionally fish and seafood, very rich, everything rich, rich, rich."

"Ice cream and stuff," explains Alan. "Although I never liked desserts. I was for meat and potatoes. I always thought breakfast was the best meal, still do. And I never drank coffee. I did smoke, cigars and pipes, but no cigarettes, never cigarettes."

The typical American diet the Keisers speak of, despite its powerful negative effects on contemporary society, was a long time coming. Initially tree people, early man ate mostly leaves and berries and nuts. The process of eating, however pleasurable or unsatisfying, essentially boils down to digestion—the effective processing of the food we eat—of which an essential element is our complex of digestive enzymes. Eventually, over many years, the cells of our ancestors developed the proper enzymes for breaking down plant carbohydrates and the few unsaturated fats found in seeds and nuts. Later, civilization evolved into two primary modes of life-style and diet—the farmer-gatherers, who stayed in one place, tended crops and ate primarily grains supplemented by dairy products, and the hunter-nomads, who moved from place to place and relied primarily on a diet of animal protein. Eventually, as civilization progressed and man moved further and further from the direct source of his food supply, he began to incorporate both dairy products and animal protein, varying his diet but greatly increasing his intake of cholesterol and saturated fat.

The animal protein, though different from that of plants, would probably not have caused undue strain on the human digestive process. It was the fat that caused the problem. Even cooked, our digestive system is unable to completely break down saturated animal fat, so the body stores what's left in what are called low-density molecules that circulate in the blood stream and eventually find a resting place in the small spots of debris that collect in our arteries. It's probably not stretching the ramifications of this brief historical vignette to suggest that the type of diet the Keisers once ate, and millions of other Americans still consume, grossly overloads the human digestive process, meaning the more fat we eat, the more waste must be disposed of— which increases the deposits along the lining of the walls of our arteries.

Although these exact thoughts undoubtedly were not on the Keisers' mind as Alan began experiencing his heart problems, both Bea and Alan were aware that certain factors had been implicated in heart disease— primarily smoking, lack of exercise, stress and a high-fat diet, although, especially at the time of Alan's first attack, the exact correlation between dietary fat and cholesterol had not been conclusively identified. After Alan's angiogram, and on the advice of their cardiologist, the Keisers attempted some modification of their diet, reducing fat intake, such as cheeses, and trying not to eat food prepared with excess fat—although Bea says there was really "no clear-cut direction." It must be remembered, however, that this was more than twenty years ago, and the idea of post–heart attack rehabilitation was not nearly as sophisticated as it is today.

Bea reminds Alan, "After the first heart attack, you stopped smoking cigars."

"That's right," Alan replies, "and I then begged the doctor to let me smoke a pipe after a while. In fact, I smoked a pipe until the second attack." As far as exercise was concerned, Bea says her husband was a golfer, "but that was it—golf and bowling."

"It was a sedentary life," concedes Alan. "When I was young, I was in good shape. And in the Army I was in good shape."

When I ask him if the first heart attack helped motivate him to change his life-style, Alan answered truthfully, "No, it took more than that."

"Alan goes in periods," explains Bea, "not that I'm not that way too. There are times when the slightest thing will make him terribly upset and it will be, 'Don't pick on me, don't try to tell me what to do.' I had to learn how to handle Alan so we could work together. And it was really the pick-and-find method, because there was nowhere to go, nobody to talk to. I did not know one person who had been in the same situation."

Alan laughs and agrees. "All I heard was 'How can a guy like you have a heart attack? You're the easiest-going guy in the world.' That was my outward appearance, I guess, to everybody."

"They used to call him grouchy and grumpy—"

"But that was at the office; to the outside world I was Mr. Nice Guy."

"That's because he was tired, he was so tired from all the work he put in."

"I used to go to sleep in the chair every night. Even if we had company, I didn't care, I fell asleep."

"That's why Alan was so easygoing," Bea laughs. "He was tired. He didn't want to fight."

I asked Bea if after the first attack she feared that Alan might have another. "I would say it's like anything else; it always stays in the back of your mind," she answers. "But it's something that's not paramount. I guess it's something like I'm left-handed and if you asked me if I'm left-handed I'll say yes, but I'm not going to go around telling you about it." So it was that when Alan had his second attack on the plane, Bea was not completely unprepared. "I did take CPR and I had a Red Cross course when I was in the scouts," she explains, "not necessarily because of Alan's problem, but it was in the back of my mind." Alan, however, contends he never worried about having another attack. "I figured if I worried about it, it's worse," he rationalizes, "so why worry about it?"

Alan's remark symbolizes a prevalent attitude among heart attack victims and characterizes a form of denial of their problem. Bea, however, expresses a different opinion. "It's an interesting thing—and stop me if you think I'm wrong now," she says to her husband, "because we've never discussed this—but I think that Alan's feeling was that it was my responsibility and not his—to see that he was all right and everything was OK. I don't know, Alan . . ."

"Could be, could be," Alan answers dispassionately, and then he admits, "I never even bothered to find out why I had a heart attack or what was wrong with me. Or what all this baloney was about— catheterizations and everything else. I never cared. I figured, 'You want to do it, do it.' And of course," he adds, "I knew she was taking care of things. She's always known as doctor. Our son Billy'll tell you who's the doctor in this house."

But Bea wants to pursue her first point. "I think that had something to do with it. But I think that Alan just thought, 'Well, it's not my problem because I know Bea's going to be there.' " Alan doesn't comment any further, except to shrug his shoulders, as if indicating, "Could be, so what?"

After Alan's first "flukey" incident, life seemed to go on as usual for the Keisers—with a few variations—until Alan began to slowly creep back toward an overloaded schedule and his former hectic pace. Bea characterizes Alan as being "heavily back to work by the time he had his second attack." Alan had, however, modified his routine somewhat and showed no further signs of heart disease until the second attack on the airplane, which set into motion a series of incidents that almost cost Alan Keiser his life.

II

"Look, in my condition, you'd better take care of it."

"The first heart attack had caused complete closure of one of the three major arteries to the heart. With the second it was not quite complete closure, but almost." Bea Keiser is describing Alan's condition after his second heart attack. "This was not blockage from cholesterol," she explains, "but a result of the heart attacks. Of course the reason he had the attacks to begin with was probably related to cholesterol deposits.

"We came home from Omaha," she continues, "and he seemed to be stabilized. He started back to work, started going in a couple of hours a day. He was tired but he was slowly going to build it up to an entire day. He was trying to get up to capacity, figuring this attack would be like the last one and he would be back to work without any complications.

"Then—I would say it was the end of January, almost a year later—Alan had an incidence of not feeling well. It happened in the middle of the night—an emergency—and we took him to the closest hospital, where he stayed for two and a half weeks while they monitored him. Because of the hospital's policies, his own doctor wasn't able to treat him—in an emergency, the doctor who admits you becomes your physician. And even though we had another cardiologist in another hospital, he was not allowed to come in and see him because he wasn't on staff. Dr. Likoff felt that Alan shouldn't be moved and that maybe he wouldn't be there that long. He was wrong," she says dryly, plowing up old ground. "Unfortunately Alan had a cardiac arrest in the hospital."

(Cardiac arrest is the result of an immediate instance of rapid heart rate. Its specific causes are unknown, but it can happen to anyone, even an individual with no history of heart disease. Most sudden deaths from heart attacks, in fact, are due to cardiac arrest. In Alan's case, given his history, there would have been a possibility that he might experience irregularities in his heartbeat that might lead to such a complication. Victims of cardiac arrest are resuscitated by electric shock.)

Alan lets go with another one of his mood-disturbing chuckles and then proceeds to tell his version of the story. "I remember we were watching TV," he says. "Bea and I and my son. And all of a sudden I turned to her and I said, 'Bea, the set is spinning; something's happening.' I passed out, I guess, and they told me afterward that I'd had a cardiac arrest."

In her understated way, Bea explains that she could see "we were definitely going to have a problem" and told Billy to run out in the hall and get help. "Then," she says, "I turned to Alan. First I gave him mouth-to-mouth resuscitation, then I gave him oyxgen and then more mouth-to-mouth. Then they came in with all the equipment."

"Machines," says Alan.

"And we were able to bring him around," sighs Bea.

"Then it was the intensive care again and then slowly getting back to some kind of stability again. Dr. Likoff still couldn't take care of him because he wasn't on staff at the hospital where Alan was, so I arranged for his associate, who lived in the area, to come visit as my brother. He would read Alan's charts in intensive care . . ."

Alan laughs and shakes his head, "The politics of medicine."

"He would tell me and I would talk to the doctor who was taking care of Alan. I'm sure Alan's physician wondered where I was getting this technical information." Bea laughs as she tells the story, but you can't help admiring the ingenuity of her ploy—and the fact that she was able to convince both Alan's cardiologist and his associate to go along with it.

"The minute we were allowed to be discharged, we took Alan by ambulance to the hospital where Dr. Likoff was," continues Bea. "Alan stayed there for more evaluation and another catheterization. What they told us when we were together was that he didn't need to have open heart [bypass] surgery." She hesitates for a moment and then says, "What they told me privately was that he couldn't have surgery because he had two arteries that were completely closed, plus a lot of scar tissue from the heart attacks. What they said," she summarizes, "was that Alan had lost a lot of his heart muscle, that all he had left was maybe thirty percent. Maybe just twenty-five to thirty percent, which meant there was no chance that he could have open-heart surgery. This was 1973."

(The damage caused to the heart muscle by a heart attack such as Alan Keiser experienced does not heal well and becomes scar tissue instead of usable muscle. Alan had had so much damage to his heart that it appeared there were no healthy areas to direct bypasses to. As one physician put it, you can't do bypass unless the heart has healthy areas of muscle remaining.)

The recitation of complications continues. Although Bea has obviously gone over this territory before, she doesn't elaborate on how she felt at the doctor's frank assessment of Alan's health. The heart, when all is said and done, is a muscle and like all muscles in the human body has a specific function and purpose. Given such large-scale damage to such an essential organ, it's easy to speculate on the negative ramifications of Alan Keiser's condition . . . and prognosis. What is normal, after all, when your heart has been reduced to less than one-third capacity?

But Bea's thoughts traveled a different byway. "If the doctors knew Alan would not survive open-heart surgery at that point," she says, "I knew that he couldn't survive another winter, that he couldn't survive the cold weather. He had to have exercise, so we had put in a pool. He was to swim every day and do some walking. Then we thought about putting a bubble over the pool so he could swim during the winter. But I thought the bubble was too experimental," she acknowledges somberly. "So I knew the only thing to do was to take him to a place where the climate would be better. We had a neighbor who had moved to Palm Beach and I thought that would probably be the place to go. And so I brought Alan down here with three of the four children with the idea that they could finish their schooling here. When we first came down we all lived in an apartment. My oldest had just finished high school."

Alan takes up the story. "Our oldest daughter didn't come down with us, she stayed up there. The rest of the kids came with us and went to school here. Then we'd go back for the summer to our home in Philadelphia. We did that for three years.''

"But I could see," says Bea, sitting cool and poised, "that in order for us to really function as a family, going back to our house up north and living in an apartment complex down here was not the best environment for children. We needed more of a sense of permanence. So we sold our house in Philadelphia and bought this house."

"And we lived here permanently," reflects Alan. "Smartest move we ever made." Then he explains how he and Bea worked to make it possible. "After '73," he says, "when I had the cardiac arrest in the hospital, I didn't go into the office anymore. We built an office in our home and I stayed home. I only went in once in a while. I did all my business on the phone."

"One thing we did in changing life-styles," Bea describes matter-of-factly, "was to take the children's playroom and turn it into Alan's office. When we came back from Omaha after the second attack, Alan said, 'What am I going to do? How are we going to handle it?' I said, 'Alan, you have to look at where you function the best. You're an executive; you have executive ability and you have expertise that no one in the business has. So now you have to use it.' The thing I used to always complain about with Alan was that he would do things that were foolish—he would spend time needlessly when a clerk in the office could be doing the same work."

"But," Alan adds playfully, "nobody could do it as good as me."

"I think that was part of the reasoning," says Bea.

"I had to learn to delegate. Now," he says humorously, "I'm overly delegating." We each grant him a small smile, and Bea continues her story. "So we took the playroom and made that into an office and got Alan a direct line. I said, 'Rather than go into your office, where if you wanted to talk to someone you could either jump up or else push a button, this way you'll only push the button.' "

"All I had to do was dial two or three numbers and somebody else would pick it up," says Alan.

"And that worked very well," concludes Bea. "If there were things Alan had to have, someone would drop them off. Alan could view them and I or someone else would take them back. So Al was able to do his work without the pressures of being at the office."

In this way, the Keisers developed an enlightened and ingenious solution to the challenge of lowering stress, a prescription recommended to most heart patients. Their ingenuity, however, was made possible in part by the fact that Alan was employed in a family-owned business.

Neither admits so directly, but the seriousness of Alan's condition must have impressed them both—to make such a dramatic change in circumstances, especially given Alan's previously expressed enthusiasm for his work.

I asked Bea and Alan if they considered Alan's pace at the office an important component of his heart attacks—whether they thought he worked under a great deal of stress.

Bea is quick to answer. "Yes," she says, "and Nathan [Pritikin] and I argued about that. I feel as if it was a very, very important part of Alan's problems. To me, stress is a kettle of boiling water going bub, bub, bub and unless you take the lid off and let the steam get out . . . it boils over. And there are ways of coping," she continues. "You have to cope with it in the way that there's the least amount of wear and tear on your own body. That's my feeling. Alan's coping skills in his office were not very good." By Alan's own admission, however, work was not the only stress with which he had to cope. "Oh, hell," he says, "I was worried about getting to the airport on time. I'd sit in the airport for four hours waiting for the airplane. Something might come up, so I'd better be there early."

Bea agrees, "It was self-imposed stress." Then she adds, "Now, the interesting thing is that in problems that we've had with our kids—that have been anywhere from mild to horrible—I marvel at Alan taking it like water off a duck's back. I absolutely marvel at the way he does that. He's taught me a little bit, but I don't know how he's been able to handle it."

"Well," Alan begins, in self-defense, "Bea was always into everything. She'd dive in and try and fix it. Which was OK," he admits. "It was right in a way. But in the same vein, I thought that if the kids were going to do things, they were going to do them whether we liked them or not, so why worry about them?" Alan's voice has dropped and changed from the lighthearted tone of an easy raconteur to the responsible voice of a parent. "If it happens, it happens," he says. "And it did happen. The kids used to drive me . . ."

Bea stops him, anticipating his conclusion. "But they didn't really drive him nuts," she says. "That's the thing I always marveled at. To me, it was like the end of the world, and meanwhile Alan might decide he wanted no part of it and he'd go to bed."

But Alan admits that if Bea weren't taking care of it, he would have to. "I'd have to do it," he says, and then adds incidentally, "Well, I can take some credit; sometimes I come up with the next move." Bea offers no comment.

Remembering their previous comments, I wondered if Alan's attitude has anything to do with wanting to be a nice guy. Bea maintains it does, and Alan admits, "Oh, with the kids, always. They could get anything they wanted from me. I was Mr. Nice Guy and she was the heavy. Then I wised up—after seeing the toll it was taking on Bea."

But Bea contends a lot of it was her own fault: "Because I felt as if 'Gee, I won't burden Alan with this,' and Alan liked what was happening, so it was easy to encourage me to continue. He was kind of feeding me a subtle message of 'Look, in my condition, you better take care of it'—not that he said it in those words."

Alan laughs thinly in the background, as if implying, "Look what I did."

Bea continues, however, seeming to regard this as an important thought. "When years later, we were finally at the Pritikin Longevity Center, one thing we learned was that it was up to Alan. I remember one of the doctors said to me something or other about a routine to take care of myself. And I said to him, 'I'm here for my husband.' And he said, 'But you're here to take care of yourself and he's here to take care of himself. And the sooner he learns that and the sooner you learn that, the better it will be.'

"I remember he said, 'It's up to you; let your husband take care of himself and you start taking care of yourself.' " Bea is quiet, momentarily thoughtful. "And it suddenly dawned on me that there I was being responsible for two people instead of just one. I'm still learning every day that Alan must take care of himself, that he must be the keeper of his own mind and body just as I have to be the keeper of my own mind and body, and it's not fair to impose my will on him. Not that Alan ever tried to impose his will on me.

"So," she summarizes, "that was the beginning of Alan assuming responsibility. 'You want to be on this diet? You're going to do it.' "

Alan agrees with her recollection. "You want to go eat ice cream and cake, go ahead and go sit in the chair again. That was always in my mind," he says seriously. "That if I ate ice cream and cake and all the other junk that I always ate, I was going to be back in this chair again where I was before we went to Pritikin."

Despite the insights they express as they review past events, Bea remembers when times were different. "The kids would come home from school and it would be 'Shish, shish, shish, Dad's sleeping.' " She leans forward in her chair and puts her finger up to her lips as if she's slipping from one room of the house to another, urging the children to be quiet. "But where was Dad sleeping?" she asks and quickly answers her own question. "Dad was sleeping in the living room."

"On the couch," Alan says, smiling as he shrugs.

"So," says Bea, "the whole house stopped."

"Not in the bedroom," laughs Alan, "nah, nah." His chuckle ripples with the wisdom of hindsight.

"What he should have done," says Bea, "if he wanted quiet, was to go into the bedroom and close the door and let the rest of the house function normally. But everybody had to be very quiet and 'shish, shish, shish,' and go off in different directions and not bother Dad because he was right there in the living room taking his nap. But you see all these things later, not initially," she concedes.

Asked whether she and the family felt any antagonism at such mannerisms, Bea answers, "We were just so happy that he was here and was functioning and he was moving forward. Our attitude was 'We'll adjust to whatever Alan is. He's the focal point for all of us.' We were all these spokes coming out from Alan. That was it."

Pushing further I wondered if the kids resented that. Bea says, "Oh yes, oh yes. None of them has really voiced it, but they've acted it out. Our oldest was going to camp—the first time she was ever away from us. She was nine years old. She was a very outgoing, warm, sharing child. We were scheduled to see her for visiting day. Instead we were in the hospital because Alan had his first heart attack. And so she had Visiting Day, the first time she was away from home, with nobody there. Friends of ours went and they played surrogate parents for the day."

"But," says Alan, "she didn't forget it."

"It's interesting that each of the things that have happened to us," says Bea with the impassivity of understatement, "have been when we have been away from home. So now the kids don't seem to want to be physically away from us. They really don't. On the other hand, I think there has been the positive part of having a physical problem—that they're more keenly aware of their own bodies."

As the Keisers speak, it's not illogical to wonder what Bea's attitude has been, caught between the dual proposition of caring for an obviously ill husband and attempting to nourish a healthy atmosphere for a growing family—a challenge that might seem to be a conflict in priorities. One thinks of stories about children, angry at a parent for some reason and immaturely wishing something to happen to them— and then something does. Or about the child who doesn't get enough attention because there is someone sick in the house and does things to get negative attention. All kinds of problems can spring from situations in which one parent has been severely ill and might die.

"My philosophy," says Bea positively, "was always that the

children—as we used to tell them—were like links in a chain. I used to explain that we were all linked together and it was important that if one of us couldn't be there, then the others should double up. That way, we could keep good family interaction constant. If I were busy with Alan . . ." She pauses, and adds, "Alan was always first; there was never a choice—Alan was always first."

Alan agrees, "We've always been first with each other."

Bea goes on to explain what this means. "I remember when our first child was a few months old. Our pediatrician was the doctor that had delivered Alan. Our daughter would cry when I put her in her playpen, so she must have been six months old. She didn't like it, and the minute I'd leave her, she'd cry. I spoke to the doctor about it and he told me, 'Look, you have things to do, and it's important that she learn how to cry. And if Alan asks you something and the baby is crying, you should listen to Alan because he came'—I remember this vividly—he said to me, 'Alan came first. And you must always remember that. He came first and your children will come subsequently after Alan.' "

There are some rumblings from Alan during this part of the conversation, but it appears he's agreeing.

"So I would tell the children, 'Each one of you is responsible for the other one. That's why it's important if Dad and I are not here, that you must help one another. You have to feel as if the family structure is the most important. You can have all your friends, but when times get down to the nitty gritty, who stands up and who's there during the rough times? Your family.' " She stops a moment, "Maybe it's because I was an only child and this was the kind of family style that I had designed in my mind.

"So," Bea continues, "that's why Alan comes first. If it weren't for Alan and I, there wouldn't be a household, and this is a story that I've played back and forth so my children feel it—that back-to-back, each one is responsible for the other one. And as a family, they're very, very close."

I asked them if Alan's heart problems have had any particular effects on the children.

"It did something to one of our daughters," says Bea. "She changed at that point in her life. I think she was afraid she was going to lose her father. When Alan was in the hospital once, I had each of the children come separately. I gave each one a time when they could come and she was the last to come because she didn't want to see her father or be with him if he was going to die."

It's a sobering thought. The room becomes still, the only sound the low humming of my tape recorder.

It's now my turn to change the subject. I ask if Alan understood how significantly he would have to change his life-style after he came home from Omaha. Bea says she knew it, "absolutely," but Alan answers, "I think I was just starting to realize it." Then he quips, "I mean, how many more chances was I going to get?"

Bea picks up on Alan's remark. "I remember Alan was recuperating—I remember it very vividly. We were sitting in front of the fire in the living room. A friend had come over. He had had a heart attack, and Alan was telling him about what he'd learned, saying, 'Look what I've gone through, and I know how I am changing my life and I'm going to be different. This is what it's going to be like for me, and I hope you will do it too.' And Alan's friend said, 'Oh, I really didn't have a heart attack.' Alan told him, 'Don't say that, I said that too. It's important to be aware of where you are at the moment and how you got to that point. You got there because you had a problem. If you don't change, you'll continue to have problems.' " She pauses to catch her breath, the knitting needles still clicking. "It was during that time that Alan was becoming very aware. We'd experienced something in a very dramatic way. We were really scooped up and put in isolation in Omaha, and so we were able to look at our situation from afar.

"By the time I came back home," she continues, "I had already had it in my mind that we were going to take the playroom for Alan's office—so that there would be the least amount of stress, which I've always felt was one thing I tried to handle as much as I could."

"That," says Alan, "was when I started going to the store, going shopping with Bea and doing the little things, taking the kids places." He maintains he enjoyed his new way of life. "I used to call the office," he laughs "and say, 'I'll be out for a while, take my calls.' " He grins. "I'd come back and get a list of calls and I'd make them and that would be the end of it. But I wouldn't be there at six o'clock in the morning till seven o'clock at night, running. And," he adds sagely, "I found out that everything I had to get done got done. If it wasn't done by me, somebody else did it. I found out I wasn't the smartest guy in the world."

Bea listens and offers further insight. "Alan also learned it was fun to work in the kitchen," she says. "He learned it didn't mean there was something wrong with his manhood if he helped me, and that it was fun to make projects out of things. He became a very involved part of the household."

"I went from one extreme to another."

"I think the kids," says Bea, "were very pleased by it."

Along with her efforts to lighten Alan's stress-related activities,

Bea undertook to encourage her husband on an exercise program. "It was gradual," she says. "We'd walk. I would try to get Alan to walk in the mall."

"In the cold," Alan explains, "we'd drive over to the mall."

"In fact," Bea remembers, "we did that even before the mall started. Sears had built—"

"A new store," Alan says, sitting up straight in his chair.

"And it was all on one floor," laughs Bea, "so we used to— "

"I knew every department in Sears backward," Alan continues.

"We'd go up and down and in and out."

"Yeah," Alan says, "it was great."

Bea adds, "Alan was always quite athletic when he was young and then he had his golf, so the walking was fun. It helped get rid of some of his energy and he enjoyed that."

The Keisers lived for three years with Alan's office in the house and with the annual commute to Florida. Bea remembers that when they moved and left Alan's Philadelphia playroom-office behind, he was concerned about how he was going to manage things. "I told him," she says, "we'll have the phones, we'll have the office setup so it's really no problem. We'll have the same thing as we had in Philadelphia. You'll still have the mails and it'll work.' "

"It did," says Alan. "I'd go up north in the spring and the fall. That was the only time I would go, never in the cold weather. I still don't go in cold weather. And it was fine. And I was feeling fine."

Bea concurs, "Fine, he was fine."

"And they never did the bypass," says Alan, pausing, "not then."

III

"I figured if this is it, this is it."

Despite the move to Florida and despite Bea's attempts to make Alan's work situation more tolerable and less intense, in April, 1979, Alan Keiser again began having chest pains—although not long in duration. According to Bea, however, their new physician in Palm Beach told them, "I really think I've reached the end of my limit; maybe you should go up and see your doctor in Philadelphia, who has really done such a wonderful job."

"Actually he wanted us to go to Atlanta to see his man," remembers Alan, "and you called Bill Likoff and he said there was no reason to go to Atlanta. He said, 'Come up here; we've got the best heart surgeon in the world; we just hired him.' Remember that?"

Bea looks out the patio door, thinks a second and agrees, "That's right. We went up to see Bill and he said, 'Stay on the same medicine; that's fine. I think he's OK.' And with that, our doctor here in Florida said, 'I don't think he's fine. I'm very upset and I've done everything I can. I want him to possibly consider having open-heart surgery.'

"But I told him," says Bea, "that I had been told by the doctors in Philadelphia he couldn't have it."

Alan interjects, "That was 1972, '73."

Bea continues, "The doctor said, 'Well, that was in 1973 and this is 1979 and a lot has happened since then. I think at this point we maybe should look into it. I would like to have him have a catheterization in Atlanta at Emory [University School of Medicine] and maybe consider having open-heart surgery.' " Alan's reaction to this new course of events is delivered flatly: "I wasn't feeling good, so anything would be better than what I was doing."

"So I called Dr. Likoff," explains Bea, "to tell him, and he said he felt he didn't want Alan to go to Atlanta. He said to me, 'I am now the president of the hospital and I can really move mountains, and if Alan is going to have a catheterization or if he's going to go anywhere, I want it to be—' "

"In my hospital," says Alan lightly, joking at his own importance.

Bea goes on, mimicking the doctor's words. "He said, 'I just saw him and I don't think he should have surgery, but let's look. We'll put him in the hospital and do some studies. We'll give him a catheterization. We have all the records here.' And he told us then he felt bypass surgery could be a possibility. To me alone he said"—her voice becomes small and very soft as she continues to describe the conversation—"he said to me, 'Alan's time really is so short and he's not going to make it, so we have nothing to lose.' "

"Hurray for me, huh?" says Alan, as he stabs at the silence that follows Bea's remark.

But Bea doesn't react to his comment. She completes the doctor's prognosis, again in dry, hushed tones, "He told me, 'We don't think he's going to live to make it through the catheterization.' "

There isn't much to say. The three of us look mutely at each other, each attuned to the significance of the doctor's sinister prognosis. Billy's basketball game drones on faintly somewhere in the background, but in this part of the house, our thoughts hug the silence.

Nudging a question slowly forward, I ask Bea if she had any idea Alan was that ill.

"Oh, yes," she says lifelessly. "Oh, yes." Her words echo in the room as if they have been pushed off a steep cliff. Alan says, "She knew, I didn't," his own voice curiously stiff. "I was doing hardly anything," he continues quietly. "I was there, I ate my meals. I watched television and did nothing. I didn't want to work, didn't want to do anything."

Bea confirms the deterioration of his condition. "He was home, but he was just here. He had no energy, absolutely no energy. Everything was an effort." She sighs. The knitting needles are cold in her hands now. Again there is a pause; slowly she smiles dryly, without humor, and says, "Luckily we got through the catheterization."

As Bea's voice trails off, prospecting for renewed energy to continue the story, Alan says quickly, his words running together, "And then the next day, the next day they took me to surgery." Quietly, Bea returns to the conversation, her voice clear but heavy with emotion, "They canceled people because there was just . . . there was just no time. Of the three coronary arteries to the heart, he had two that were already gone."

"And the third one was—" interrupts Alan, quieter now than he has been up to this point. But his wife beats him: "And the third one was ninety-five percent blocked."

An improbable chill seems to have swept into the room, stealing beneath our thoughts. Bea says very softly—so that we must strain to hear her, "Alan was a whisper away, a whisper away." The thought hangs. "What was keeping him alive," she explains, "was that above the point where the arteries had closed there had started to develop little tiny collateral vessels. They were minor but strong enough—despite the three arteries just about closing—to keep him alive."

Collateral circulation is an established medical fact. Under demand, the major arteries of the heart generate small feeder vessels—many of them—to serve areas of the heart ordinarily nourished by the main arteries. The key, however, is that there must be demand for increased blood supply. In Alan's case, his routine of regular walking helped stimulate the growth of collateral circulation to his damaged heart. Ordinarily, bypass surgery is not recommended in individuals in whom adequate collateral circulation has been developed. But the complications of Alan's case seemed to have called for more creative medical thinking.

"You remember the doctor had told me he thought Alan had about twenty-five or thirty percent of his heart muscle left?" she asks. "Well, during the bypass surgery he lost tissue—twelve percent more—which always happens, but they don't tell you. In Alan's case, this was crucial because he had so little.''

Alan sits quietly in his chair; he doesn't comment on what Bea has said, so she continues. "So by the time he got out of surgery, Alan had fifteen percent of his heart function left. He survived the surgery because the doctor worked very, very fast. He did the work he had to do in a little less than an hour and a half—for a quadruple bypass.''

Alan chuckles ever so slightly, nervously, but still makes no comment. Bea plunges onward.

"Alan was really a pretty sick guy," she almost whispers. There is silence again. Even the ballgame seems to have faded into another dimension. In another moment, Bea repeats herself: "Alan was a pretty sick guy. They didn't know whether he was going to make it or not. Then he had every complication imaginable. He was seventeen days in intensive care.''

Bea's last words spark distasteful memories for Alan. "Can you imagine?'' he asks rhetorically. "I'll never forget that.'' His eyes blink pain at the thought. His hand reaches for his throat, he strokes it remembering. "I had such . . . things stuck down my throat,'' he says harshly. "I never . . . I was trying to yank them out.'' He imitates the motion of pulling tubes out of his mouth. "Oooh, I'll never forget that. I never want to be in intensive care again.''

I asked him if he realized the seriousness of his condition before he went into surgery. "They told me,'' he says tonelessly, "that maybe, maybe I'd come out of it.'' Before I can ask him how he felt about that, he stops me. "I went to sleep and that was it.'' I pressed and asked if he and Bea had a chance to discuss any of this. Alan answers, "Not a chance.'' But Bea explains, "He was really pretty sick,'' as if these few words explain it all. She repeats them to herself in a low, shallow voice. "He was pretty sick.''

Alan makes a vague attempt at lightening the mood. "We had no chance . . .'' But Bea suggests other possibilities."I think it was also that Alan just wouldn't discuss it. I began to see that 'Don't worry, just don't worry' was his thing. 'Don't worry, don't worry, everything will be fine.' ''

Again the house is still. Again Alan attempts to break the tension. "Well . . .'' he starts.

"Yes, I know.'' Bea nods very softly.

"Yeah,'' he says, "how many days was I in the hospital—fifty-four, sixty-four?''

"I don't know," Bea says, absently. "Yes." Then she adds, in that small, soft voice, "It was hard, it was long."

Gradually our conversation has come to a halt. For Alan, these experiences herald a time of triumph. For Bea, they represent barely expressible worry and frustration. For the first time really, her narrative skills wane. Alan, perhaps buoyed by the thought of how he cheated death, picks up the tale. "We came home though," he says firmly, netting the silence with a smile.

Slowly Bea rallies, her voice still soft. "And that's what counts," she says, as if trying to convince us all. "We came home."

"June, July wasn't it?" asks Alan. When Bea doesn't respond, he lets it lay. She doesn't seem to have anything to say.

I asked Bea if she can remember her feelings during this time. "I just, I just . . ." she begins, pauses and then picks up her thought. "You know what I did? I divided the day into thirds. I would say, 'Well, I just hope he can make it up to lunch and then we'll get . . .'"

Before she can finish, Alan says with a chuckle, "I wasn't going to leave you stuck that early, Bea."

But his wife is not easily sidetracked. ". . . and then from lunch to dinner, and then from dinner to getting to bed and getting up in the morning and then . . . So it was like I never faced the whole day. I just dealt with what I had to deal with." She pauses, brightens a little. "I will tell you a little aside funny. Actually it's not funny. The day before Alan went into surgery I called home to see how everything was and our daughter Emmy said to me, 'Oh, Mom, the worst thing just happened—they just arrested Milda.' "

"Our housekeeper," says Alan.

"So I asked her," continues Bea, " 'Why did they arrest Milda?' And Emmy said, "Oh, because she shot her lover . . .' "

Alan laughs a big laugh. "They had to give her that on top of everything else," he says. "We had to make arrangements to get her bail and everything. She said she didn't do it." He laughs again heartily.

"I had to call friends to lend money to get her out on bail, all this while Alan . . ."

"While I'm waiting for surgery."

We all laugh, glad for the break, and Bea starts to take up the story again. "Anyway, we brought Alan home . . ." But Alan seems inclined to slow the conversation. He verifies again that he came home in July. Bea confirms it and then says matter-of-factly, "Then he went into heart failure, at the end of July." I take a breath and then ask gently about the prognosis after that. Alan delivers it, somber for really the first time, "Not good."

Bea, in a very soft voice, again recalling difficult times, says, "No, not good." But," she adds wearily, "they let him go home because there was nothing else—"

Alan cuts her off, "Two months in the hospital is enough."

It's difficult to convey the fatigue with which we relive this segment of Alan's story. Ordinarily a light, cheerful woman, Bea's expression has now become tight, strained. Her words suggest frustration at the dead end to which medicine had brought them. "They couldn't do anything more," she reflects, "so they let him leave the hospital. I kept him in Philadelphia in a hotel for a few days, but Alan said, 'I want to get out of here, I want to go home.' And so I took him home to Florida, because I figured that was the best place for him to recuperate.

"At home, it was an effort for him to do much of anything. First of all, after lying almost two and a half months in the hospital, you can lose strength from just inactivity. Plus the open-heart surgery. So he had slowly to build up his strength. He was eating," she remembers, "but he really had no interest in anything. Everything was an effort. He just wasn't really responding." She adds, still weary, "Our doctor here in Palm Beach told us, 'I am at my wits' end, take him back to Philadelphia. Maybe they can do something for him up there . . . adjust the medication, maybe that's what he needs.' So we took him back to Philadelphia to see what we could do about getting him a better quality of life, so he could function a little bit better." Her empty voice recalls the futility of the trip. "They . . . they changed the medicine around" is all she says, her sentence slamming to the floor in a dull thud.

"That's when they gave us the presoline," remembers Alan. (Apresoline is a drug usually prescribed for individuals with severe hypertension.)

"Yes," says, Bea, "the presoline. And Alan came home and he felt good. Then all of sudden he started to go down, down. He was really sinking, really sinking fast."

I asked Bea, quietly, if she felt that he was dying. Without hesitation, she says emphatically, "Oh, I knew he was."

"And me," says Alan. "I felt the same way."

"How does that feel?" I asked him.

"Let me tell you," he answers, "it doesn't feel good."

"You could feel the strength leaving you?" I pressed further.

"Yeah," Alan's answer bounces back against the quiet of the

room. "I couldn't make it to the bathroom and back without someone helping me."

"It was awful," sighs Bea, who has barely moved, her elbow on the table next to her, her forehead leaning on outstretched fingers. "It was terrible. It was awful to sit there and watch him."

"That was it, that was as far as I could get," says Alan. (The distance from Alan's chair to the nearest bathroom is about ten feet.)

"Did you care?" I asked.

"Yeah, I cared," he answers, "but I was to the point that I thought, 'If this it, this is it. That's all.' "

"He gave up," says Bea, her voice a reflection of cold finality. "He really gave up."

I asked how she felt when she saw this happening.

"Well, there was something else that happened concurrently," she begins, her voice now lighter but still weary. "I was watching when Alan took his medicine, and he seemed to go pho-o-o-sh." She makes a movement with her arm, dropping it toward the floor like a dead weight and releasing all the air from her lungs. "I thought, 'Something's not right, something's not right.' Then I was talking to a girl on the telephone who was telling me about a woman who was very ill—she was eighty-five years old and very ill. She had heart failure. While she's talking to me, I was thinking to myself, 'This woman's eighty-five, and my husband's in his fifties and he's . . . and it's just not fair.' But I listened to what she said. She told me a pharmacist had reviewed the medication this woman was taking and asked if she took all of her medicine at once.

"Now, why she should tell me this," Bea continues, "when I'm really not that friendly with her before or after . . . It was just a chance conversation. But it turned out that taking the two medications together took all of the electrolytes out of the body at one time. It was robbing her of her strength, and this lady was literally dying in front of her eyes. Then she proceeds to tell me how she hates the medical profession. Finally I asked, 'What's the medication?' It turned out it was the same medication . . ."

Alan interrupts, again brandishing an air of triumph at his wife's investigative efforts, "Exact medication I was on. And I was taking it the same way."

(One of Alan's drugs was Lasix—a very powerful diuretic prescribed to reduce Alan's blood pressure and the load on his heart. Given in excessive amounts, Lasix can lead to serious water and electrolyte depletion. Electrolytes are essential salts that exist in critical percentages in the body and are carried in the blood system. In a person with heart disease, it is important to keep the sodium chloride level down and the potassium chloride level up. Too much potassium loss—in this case from the powerful diuretics he was taking—caused Alan Keiser's critical feeling of weakness.)

"Nobody told us differently," says Bea. "So now my mind goes click, click, click. I call up our local cardiologist and tell him that I'm going to have Alan take his medicines an hour apart. He says, 'OK if you want to,' and thinks I'm funny in the head. I then call the two cardiologists in Philadelphia and I tell them that I am sure this is why Alan is so weak and can't handle himself and they think, 'Funny in the head, OK? If she wants to believe that, it's OK.' Then I called a friend of ours who's a cardiologist in New York and I asked him. He's a super guy. He said, 'Look, Bea, I'm not aware of it, but if you say so, I'll check into it.' Then he called me back and said, 'Yes, with these properties, this could happen and this is probably what has happened. I will now watch all of my patients in the future and see that they will not be given these medications together.' I made the doctors in Philadelphia do the same and also the doctors here, the five cardiologists in the group. So that's five and four in Philadelphia—"

Alan provides the total: "Ten doctors."

"Yes," says Bea, "that never knew it."

"That little chance conversation," says Alan, in typical understatement, "made a lot of difference."

"That," says Bea quietly but with authority, "that saved his life."

IV

"I ate corn; I like corn, so I ate the corn and baked potatoes . . ."

With the change in Alan's medication, the Keisers experienced a temporary reprieve from what looked like an inevitable conclusion to their struggle—and with it an insight that probably did save Alan's life. I asked how long it took before they saw some improvement from Alan's new schedule of medication.

"Oh," says Alan, "I was perking up a little, but I wasn't much better."

Bea maintains, "I would say in about four or five days I started to see a change. That," she says purposefully, "made me realize that the doctors really don't know." She admits this realization made her "very angry, very angry. It went back," she says, "to that first doctor who insisted that Alan was too young to have a heart attack. And it was related to my initial feeling that I am upset with any doctor that plays God and thinks he knows it all. I'll never forget that man who was an associate of Dr. Likoff whom we met when I took Alan up there on one of our trips—in October. He was also the one who discharged Alan. At that time, I said to him something like 'I'd be very interested to know what kind of a program Alan could go on, and now that you're discharging him if I have any problems when I get home or if I run into any problems on the plane . . .' But he said to me, 'My dear lady, you don't have any problems. He doesn't have any time; so it doesn't matter.' She repeats the sentence, 'You don't have any problems because he has no time.' There is silence in the room again, this time a silence bound by the sharp edge of anger. "I told him, 'I think you're incompetent,' and I walked away.

"So," she summarizes in a tired voice, "there was absolutely nothing . . . nothing . . . no hope. Except," she says, her tone lightening, "when Alan had his bypass, there was a lady whose husband had bypass surgery the same day. She told me that her husband was very prepared for the surgery because he was on the Pritikin diet."

Alan grins slightly in anticipation of what's to come.

" 'Oh, what is that?' I asked her. So she proceeds to tell me. Nathan had just come out with his first book, *Live Longer Now*. I called and had it delivered to the hospital. I read it while Alan was in intensive care. I also remembered that a friend of the family, a cardiologist, had had dinner with Nathan Pritikin. Because basically of what Nathan had said, this doctor used a similar regimen of diet and exercise, although he doesn't call it Pritikin. He also told me that he had one patient who had really gone down every single road that Alan had, except that he wasn't a candidate for open-heart surgery. That person went to the Pritikin center in Santa Barbara. A year later they did some tests and two years later, they did a catheterization. They couldn't believe he was the same person they had seen, because it was a marked, marked improvement.

"So that was in the back of my mind," she continues. "We knew a little bit about it because we had seen the *60 Minutes* show [which had presented a one-year follow-up of patients on the Pritikin Program]. I finally asked Alan if he would consider going to Pritikin. He said no." Prompted, Alan explains himself, "Was he smarter than my doctors?" and leaves it at that.

But Bea plunges on. "Anyway," she says, "Alan was not inter-

ested. So I called our friend and asked if he would consider helping me
get to Pritikin personally . . ."

Alan interrupts, now ready to fill in background. "That was on
Thanksgiving, wasn't it, or the day before Thanksgiving?"

Bea avoids his question and continues her story. "He recommended I call Nathan directly. So I called person-to-person and Nathan
was out. Then I called again. I called three times and Nathan never
returned the call, so I called my friend back and explained to him what
was going on. He said, 'Let me call, I know Alan's history. I'll have
Nathan call you.'

"So," she continues, her words, thoughts, coming rapidly now,
"Nathan subsequently called me, and he said, 'I just got a call from your
doctor friend, who tells me that you would like to come out with
your husband.' I told him that was true. And then Nathan said, 'I think
we can help him.' I said, 'That's wonderful.' By that time I had sent
Alan's records all over the country and they had all come back with the
message that nothing could be done, that no one could help us. I had the
records flown to Texas, to DeBakey; they were sent to Chicago; they
went to Stanford, to Boston. Every answer came back saying, 'Forget
it; there's no way we can help your husband.' "

Alan breaks in with a chuckle that seems to imply 'See what a
difficult case I was,' adding a shrug of the shoulders that suggests
further, 'What did they know?'

Bea continues her story. "So I said to Nathan, 'They've told me
all over the country there's no one who can help.' Nathan said to me,
'But I didn't say I couldn't help.' Then he asked what medicine Alan
was on, and I remember taking the phone into the bathroom and
standing in front of the medicine cabinet reading everything off. He
said, 'Oh, my, that really is a very aggressive schedule of medications.
I don't know about that. But just bring your records and be out here on
Sunday.' "

Again the pregnant pause. "This was Wednesday before Thanksgiving," says Alan. Bea recalls, "They waived something because
Nathan wanted us there and we were able to get a space." Alan
continues to interject the fine points. "Friday you went to get the
records."

"I went to get the records," she agrees, "and the nurse and the
doctor said, 'Well, we wish you well because we don't know anyone
who can stay on that diet.' " Alan laughs. But Bea says, "All I was
thinking about was 'Can we get him out there?' "

Alan chuckles again, "Meanwhile . . ."

"Meanwhile Alan's family thought I was going to kill him," says

Bea with animation, "really going to kill him, taking him out there. He was so bad I had to take him out in a wheelchair."

"To the quackery," says Alan.

"All our friends thought—"

"They all thought we were crazy."

"Not one person," remembers Bea, "with the exception of our doctor friend, who encouraged me. Everybody else thought I was—"

"Cuckoo. Even Dr. Likoff," remembers Alan. "He was dead adamant against it."

"They really thought I'd flipped," concedes Bea dully. "And I remember thinking to myself, 'I know that if I keep him here he is going to die.' That I knew. I knew as sure as anything, because he wasn't getting any better. Even though I had helped with the medication, I realized the doctors didn't know everything. In fact, that was what they'd say to me: 'We can't know everything.' But I knew if I kept him here, he couldn't make it. So I thought, 'If God is good enough to allow us to get there, maybe he's been keeping Alan alive. I thought to myself, 'There's got to be a reason. There's got to be a reason, so get him out there and keep him, keep him going . . .' "

Alan predictably softens the emotion with an interjection. "Only the good die young," he says with a grin.

Bea ignores him. "I just . . . I just felt as if I just had to get him out there. And I will tell you"—as tense wire scrapes across her words—"it was a frightening thing because there wasn't one person that was really with me. It was awful."

"No support at all," agrees Alan. He adjusts himself in his chair. "I only remember getting in the big limousine when we got to California. That's all I remember."

But the trivial details remain with Bea. "I remember Alan being in a wheelchair and me running after him through the airport here because the redcap was going very fast. I was running with the luggage trying to keep up. It was awful, I'll never forget it. I thought, 'My God what am I going to do when we get to Los Angeles?' But we got him off the plane and somebody came up to us, and said, 'I'm here from Pritikin.' And I thought, 'Isn't that nice, that is really very nice.' " Her voice becomes tiny and she sighs, remembering her relief and the small kindness of a stranger. Alan growls that he wasn't that impressed that someone had come to meet them.

Bea continues, "And then when we got there to the Center . . ." But now it's Alan's time to take up the story. He seems to have something that he wants to say—as if the account has suddenly come alive for him. "What did they tell you when you went for the examination with the doctor?" he asks his wife.

"Well, first of all," says Bea, beginning at the beginning, "we couldn't take steps anywhere, and when we got out of the limousine and saw all those steps . . ." (There is a flight of shallow steps as you enter the Santa Monica Pritikin Longevity Center from the street. The steps lead up into the lobby and put you squarely at the front registration desk. There is really no other way for registering patients to conveniently enter the building.)

Alan recalls, irritation rubbing at his voice, "We had to walk up those seven or eight steps." Bea admits, "He wasn't very happy about those steps. He was very annoyed at why we were there, too." To which Alan responds, in a tone mimicking outrage, "Absolutely, she dragged me out there for what? I was so mad at her I wanted to kill her."

I asked Alan if he agreed to go, or if he fought Bea before they left.

"I told her I didn't want to go," he answers simply. "Doctors can't be all wrong."

"How did you feel?" I looked at Bea. "Were you ready to crack?"

"Oh yes, oh yes," she answers, and then adds, "but there wasn't time." Alan says pensively, "There must have been something in the back of my head because I never did ever put my papers in order or anything like that, figuring that I was going somewhere. There had to be something in the back of my mind."

"Interesting," adds Bea, "because during the whole time, all those years and problems, this was the one time that Alan's affairs were not in order. And, God forbid, had anything happened . . ."

Alan brushes it off. "No way," he says, as if he would never have been so irresponsible, and he moves to push the conversation forward, "So we got to Pritikin . . ."

Bea says, "We got there and we went to see the doctor they had assigned us to. Alan went for his first blood test. I remember he was upset because he had to go at six o'clock in the morning. He was very upset, but we went." Bea pauses, moves her legs a bit, her sandals brushing the tile floor. "We got to the doctor," she recalls. "We were sitting across from him. He had Alan's charts and everything. We were sitting there and he looked up and said to us, 'I'm just going through your records, Mr. Keiser, and if I had seen these records before, I never would have let you come.' "

Silence again, a thin, shrill silence. Alan says dully, "That's right."

But Bea quickly continues, completing the interchange. " 'I would never have let you come, Mr. Keiser,' " she repeats, " 'because we can't help you.' " She pauses, speaks again, slowly. "Sitting there, I thought, I just thought . . . the whole world went askew. I saw a big hole and Alan going right down into it."

Alan picks up the thread, projecting his own voice as that of a spoiled child, "I said to Bea, 'All right, see, let's go home.' "

But Bea wasn't finished. "I said to the doctor, 'Well, you said you can't help him . . .' "

Alan finishes her question, " 'But can you hurt him?' " He looks directly at his wife. "That's just what you said: 'You can't help him but can you hurt him?' "I guess," he says, looking my way, "they decided they couldn't, but they treated me with kid gloves when they took me down to the treadmill."

Bea reminds him, "You were upset; remember how upset you were? First of all," she explains, "he only lasted ten seconds on the treadmill."

"Ten seconds, that was it," says Alan. "So they gave me a program for the first two weeks of five minutes on the treadmill at the slowest speed it could go. I was hooked up with doctors standing around and nurses monitoring me on the treadmill and the whole smear—and then I spent five minutes sitting in the chair, for fifteen minutes each. That was my exercise program for the day."

When I asked him what he thought about the Center and what they served him to eat, Alan answers emphatically, "Oh, I wouldn't eat that food." Bea describes him as "a complainer. He was terrible."

"I ate corn," says Alan. "I like corn so I ate corn and potatoes. I didn't even like the bread. I had a banana . . ."

"You hated the smell of the bread," Bea reminds him.

"Our room," Alan explains, "was above the kitchen and you smelled that tomato-sauce smell. That cook made everything with tomato sauce. It was horrible, the bedclothes smelled of it, the room smelled of it. Everything smelled of that goddamned Pritikin smell; that's what I still call it."

"But," observes Bea, "after the second week, we sort of got together with one of the therapists, and we said, 'We're getting nowhere. Let's get Alan on the treadmill and try it for a little longer. Let's speed it up a little and see what we can do.' " She says this in a very conspiratorial voice. "And we developed a whole new program. The therapist told the doctors about it and they told us there was no way they'd let him do it.''

"But," Alan remembers, "we said we'd be responsible for it."

Bea continues slowly but now enthusiastically, "And within a week, we were starting to walk. We made the pier—what was it, the end of the third week?" she asks Alan and then doesn't wait for an answer. "We made the pier and back. And after the fourth week, we were walking toward the Venice pier. We got down to the Venice pier [about two and a half-miles from the center] and then we took a cab back."

Alan, becoming animated, corrects her, "No, no, we took the bus back. For me, that was a new life," he acknowledges. "And we found the Boulangerie around the corner so I could eat some soup that tasted half decent and the bread. Every day that's all I did, I stuffed bread into my face—that sourdough. I weighed 139 pounds. I looked like I just got out of a concentration camp. Once we got home, we started to walk here, and we've been walking every single day since then, four to five miles."

I ask Alan whether initially he felt any better at the center and whether—as is sometimes the case—the doctors weaned him off his medication.

"No," he says, "the doctors was scared to death to tamper with me."

"In fact," Bea remembers, "I wanted to order a treadmill so we could have it at home. They wouldn't let me order it because they didn't think Alan had the stamina for it. They didn't give us the OK to order the treadmill until the fourth week. It was really something. One of the doctors told us, 'I never thought that he would ever, ever, do what he's doing.' "

There is silence again, this time the silent pride of accomplishment. Alan completes his triumph. "I called my doctor here," he says, "before we came home and I told him, 'I'm bringing the records with me because I want you to see them.' He asked me how I was doing. I told him, 'Oh, I've just walked a few miles.' He said, 'What?' 'Yeah, just walked a few miles,' I told him, 'and feel great.' He didn't believe me, he really didn't. But from the day we came back and I took those records over, that whole office has been recommending Pritikin, having people call us all the time to give advice on what to do and how to do it."

I wanted to know if he felt any better before he and Bea suggested the accelerated exercise program. "I really don't know," Alan answers.

"I was feeling so ill. I was sitting around. I was reading, I was doing nothing."

I asked if he was scared.

"Scared," he admits.

Bea characterizes it for him, "Fear and anxiety. And anger at being there, anger . . ."

Alan says again, "The food was so horrible."

Bea explains further, "I think it was anger with what had happened to him. I think everything caught up to him and he was very angry."

"Yeah," Alan agrees, "finally."

"And he was very belligerent," adds Bea. "He was not nice to people." She looks at her husband, "You were not nice to people." Again Alan agrees. "But the last two weeks," he reminds her, "I made up for it, I sure did. We were there for the full twenty-six days," he continues, "and I was walking almost five miles when we left, although we weren't going too fast. There was a man who was in the same boat I was—almost. And he had to walk like me—shuffling. So his wife and Bea used to walk ahead, and he and I would walk behind them. And he would sit down and wait for me to come back and pick him up again— because he couldn't walk as far as I was going."

"Did seeing the other people at the center give you any perspective on the degree of your own illness?" I asked Alan.

"In the beginning," he answers, "I was an outcast. I had to do the five-minute bit on the treadmill. Everybody else was walking, going all over the place. They were jumping around having themselves a gay old time and here I was doing nothing, but after a while, after we got in with the groups . . ."

Bea interrupts him, "That was where the anger was"—and Alan concurs—"because he wasn't part of the group, and all of his life he's been sort of part of the group. In one of the gatherings at the center, we met a woman named Mary Tarzian who had come with her husband, Sarcus. For some reason whatever I said hit her and she was very moved by it."

"She stuck to Bea like glue," says Alan.

"Anyhow," Bea goes on, "one day after she had come back from seeing one of the doctors, she repeated their conversation to our whole group. The doctor had said to her, "Now, don't expect any miracles here, Mrs. Tarzian.' And she said to him, 'On the contrary, doctor,' she said, 'I have just met one.' She meant Alan," confides Bea. "Although we started out by being on the outside, he was the hero of the whole center, the hero of our group." As if to clarify her point, Bea explains, "There were a lot of very seriously ill people at the center. It was the

Last Chance Motel. Alan really personified most of the people. I remember one woman had glaucoma, and her glaucoma was helped. It was like going to Lourdes and seeing these miracles.''

So Alan Keiser went home once more. This time, he had something to go on. Through the persistent efforts of his wife, he had another chance at life. And he took it. Alan is now formally retired. His brother bought out his half of the business they founded together, although Alan continues to serve as a consultant to the company. Today, his days are full and busy with the kind of community work he and Bea love. Alan presently serves as a director on the board of a local Palm Beach savings and loan association, of which he was a founder and where he also functions as chairman of the audit committee. He is also active in the Rotary, and, like Bea, he works for a variety of charitable organizations. "Plus," he says, "I've got my needlepoint, my reading. There's plenty to do." Plenty to do includes walking four to five miles a day at a brisk pace, usually in the morning. Bea joins him on his walks and Alan facetiously complains that she still beats out a better pace than he. The Keisers also golf together regularly and travel extensively, often visiting friends in various parts of the country. Alan has reduced the stock of medications formerly overflowing his medicine cabinet to continued doses of Lasix to help eliminate excess fluids and lighten the load on his heart. He still carries the nitroglycerin pills in his pocket but has not used any since his second heart attack on the plane between Los Angeles and Philadelphia. He monitors his cholesterol regularly and is satisfied that it's in reasonable limits, which in Alan's case routinely runs a little over 200. Concerned that this was too high, given his history, Nathan Pritikin and the Keisers had at one time worked out a plan to lighten the dosage of Lasix. Under the supervision of his Palm Beach physician, Alan gradually decreased his dosage. Although his cholesterol did drop, Alan reports that he was not feeling as well and has opted to continue with the originally prescribed dosage.

As they describe it, the Keisers eat out regularly, in local restaurants or at formal functions related to the various community organizations in which they serve. Their four children are grown and are busy in their own lives, but as Bea says, their children still want to be close, and the links of the Keiser family chain remain strong and supportive. Altogether, it is far from the life you might imagine for a man who has survived three heart attacks, cardiac arrest, heart failure and a quadruple bypass.

Alan Keiser was lucky. He challenged time, and—with the commitment of his wife, Bea—he beat it. Now it's his own spirit that keeps him winning against supposedly unbeatable odds. His is a full and rewarding life. Most of all, it is a life of considerable exhilaration and joy.

Some Keiser Words to the Wise

When the Keisers returned to Florida, the alumni coordinator at the Pritikin Longevity Center in Santa Monica asked if they would be willing to help establish a Pritikin support group in their area. After an initial meeting at their home, Alan and Bea and the fledgling group decided to meet regularly in restaurants and were successful in influencing a number of local establishments to develop Pritikin menus. The Keisers offered to share insights gained from their efforts with the alumni groups and from Alan's experiences on the Pritikin Program.

Both Alan and Bea have definite opinions of the benefits of having an understanding spouse.

Bea explains, "I always go along with Alan rather than have him be the odd man out, the one with the two heads. When the two of us do it, people ask, 'What are you doing? Why are you eating that way?' And I say, 'It's fun.' Usually they're bulging out of their dresses or else they can't eat, and they just say, 'Oh,' and forget it. But we have had people respond, 'Gee wiz, maybe I ought to go on that diet.' Then we explain, 'It's not a diet, it's a way of life.'

"This is a very social town," she continues, "but everything essentially centers around the Breakers. We have at least one formal affair a week there. When we go, we just call and say, 'We'll have the Keiser dinner,' which is spaghetti with tomato sauce and a sliced apple for dessert. There are always rolls on the table, which we eat without butter. There's always salad, and they serve it separately from the dressing, so we can put on a drop or not or whatever we want. So there's really no problem as far as handling ourselves."

Alan supports her thought. "That's the thing," he says, "to make it a life-style."

"And semantics is very, very important," says Bea. "I think it's the way you talk about what you're doing and the example you set. Alan has become an example. He is on the program and lives the life-style because it works well for him, but he also knows people are watching him. So as a result, he knows he has an obligation to fulfill. I'm speaking for Alan," she reflects, "when I say that, but I think it makes him feel good . . . that what he is doing and what he has been through have not been in vain. That everyone, including himself, has gained tremendously by it.''

Reinforced by Alan, she adds another thought about commitment to life-style change. ''Everybody has to pick a number that is right for them, a percentage of adherence to the diet—a percentage they'll live with for the rest of their life. Alan says his is between seventy-five and eighty percent. And whatever the person chooses, he or she has to learn to put it in the right perspective. It was Dr. Bauer at the Miami Pritikin center who helped with that. He said, 'You can bend the rule and bend the rule and pretty soon you're going in the opposite direction until you're going backward. So when you bend the rule, you have to realize how far you're bending it. If it's only a little bit and you're back on course, that's fine, but if you keep on bending it . . . it will break.' ''

Bea continues, ''I know I went on the program initially because it was easier to do, and because I didn't want to go back to living my old life-style. Intellectually I knew when I ate meat it was not the best thing for me. Now everytime I eat something that I shouldn't, it registers back here in my computer. Maybe I will eat a couple of things and start to go like this . . .'' She demonstrates a backward curve. ''But I always go back. It never goes all the way around.''

When I asked Bea how she felt when she was counseled at the Pritikin center to look after her own health and allow Alan to do the same, she answers, ''I was relieved. I thought to myself, 'I now don't have to tell Alan what he should or should not eat, what he should do, because he's learning intellectually and emotionally.' At the center, they dealt with all the various component parts—food, exercise, attitude—and it added up to make sense. And he was beginning to feel better. So rather than my saying, 'Alan should you eat this or Alan should you do that,' he himself began to see this is what he should do.''

Musing about the role of serious illness in enforcing adherence to a change in life-style, Alan Keiser grants, ''It's the biggest thing. People ask me, 'How do you have such will power that you don't eat desserts?' I tell them, 'Because I have a picture in my mind of sitting in that chair and not being able to make it to the bathroom. I don't want to do that again, so I don't want to eat these desserts and have that problem. I don't want to take that chance.' ''

As if to illustrate, Alan describes his restaurant habits. ''Always a salad,'' he says, ''and a baked potato or two baked potatoes or a bowl of soup—if it's salty I just don't eat it. I used to ask for tastes, but I decided the hell with it. For the two bucks or two-and-a-half bucks it costs for a bowl of soup, if the damn thing is salty, I'll just leave it. I won't eat crazy soup like split pea with ham or with hot dogs, but regular split pea is fine. And gazpacho; I could eat two or three bowls of gazpacho for dinner and forget about the meal.''

"One of the things that I think is really important is not to look at the menu," suggests Bea.

"Any good restaurant will make you what you want," Alan maintains. "We went to a big dinner the other night where they had roast beef. The Hyatt hotel doesn't vary, which means we couldn't order anything special. So we got a fruit plate.''

"We watched the people watching us," laughs Bea. Then she adds another thought, "We try to stay away from new and different restaurants unlesss we can't avoid it. Even then we find there's no problem.''

"For example," says Alan, "we were talking tonight of maybe going to a little Mexican restaurant. I'll get a quesadilla with no cheese. For me, they'll put in those little scallions and green pepper and mushrooms. It'll be dry but it will be gorgeous. Then I'll get a chicken taco with no cheese. It will have the lettuce and tomato, chopped up with onions and a little bit of chicken. Maybe it will have a little bit of grease or something in it—I don't know—but there won't be that much. That's what I'll have for dinner, and it'll be fine.

"You know what bothers me about eating with other people?" he suddenly asks. "When they all whisper about what they're going to order. I tell them, 'Order what you want. You want to eat a steak? That's your problem not mine.' They wait, and then ask what I'm ordering. I'll say, 'I'm ordering spaghetti with a plain tomato sauce full of garlic.' And they'll answer, 'Well, we don't like the garlic.' 'Then,' I say, 'order it without the garlic.' Sometimes they decide to try it and they find out it's not that bad.''

I wanted to know from Alan if coping with heart disease is a constant problem, something from which he never escapes.

"It's there, that's all," he observes, and then adds, with typical Keiser good humor, "The only time I make a big deal out of it is when we're at a party and it's boring. At nine or nine-thirty, after we've had dinner and they're sitting around boring everybody to death, I'll say, 'Bea,' and she'll nod, 'OK.' And then I announce, 'In my condition I have to be in bed early.' Everyone understands. Everybody's sympathetic—'he's a sick man.' '' He laughs heartily. "I look sick, don't I? That's what I used to do when I was lecturing for Pritikin. I'd ask the audience, 'Do I look sick? This is what Pritikin does.' You've got them in the palm of your hand.''

He continues, "We were discussing the 100 percent business before. I remember at one of the Pritikin alumni meetings, somebody made the statement that anybody that stays on this thing 100 percent is the guy who will fall off it the quickest. It's true. The ones that acclimate themselves to the best they can get and still keep their numbers within reason, they're the ones that can stay on the program forever."

Bea adds, "Rigidity. It's the rigidity that frightens people. I used to do a tremendous amount of cooking," she reflects. "Whenever we traveled, I would always buy a cookbook. It's a fun thing to do. It packs easy, it's not expensive and you have a nice memento. At first it was not easy cooking Pritikin, but I did creative cooking. I don't use the recipes. What I do for Alan and me is that I always have chicken soup on hand. I learned something from Madame Wu, who owns Madame Wu's in Los Angeles. If you have chicken stock—ours is always defatted—and put it to the boil once a week, it stays indefinitely.

"So I always have a pot of chicken soup in my refrigerator," she says, "and in twenty minutes I can make a dinner from the chicken soup. I'll just heat up the broth with noodles or with rice. Also I can put in matzo balls, which I always have in the freezer. Or I will take the chicken soup and puree leftover vegetables with a little bit of yogurt and I have a cold soup, very fast, one, two, three. You can take tomatoes if you want and add a little milk to it and you have either hot or cold tomato soup garnished with a little of the fresh tomato. Or I'll use some of the chicken stock and sauté some onions in it to make Alan an onion omelette or eggs and onions, with egg whites and Egg Beaters.

"And when we're entertaining, I make something for Alan and something else for our guests so they don't feel as if, 'Oh my goodness, we're going there and they're going to give us Pritikin food.' "

Alan pipes up, "Yeah, so people don't have to think they'll have to eat that food."

"But it's amazing," she continues, "how many things I make that can be OK for Alan. Like I'll make mussels marinara sometimes and I will make a delicious chicken dish with onions and green peppers that's absolutely superb. There are all kinds of dishes. Once you realize what the real culprits are, all you have to do is substitute. And if you can put it out so it looks pretty, that really helps very much."

When they travel, the Keisers frequent Italian or Chinese restaurants and order the food prepared the way they want. "Or sushi," says Alan. "I love sushi."

It looks like Alan Keiser will have the last word. He sits back in his chair and takes a sip of the pink lemonade Bea has brought him. "I still walk behind her all the time," he says. "She's still faster than I am." Then he thinks the thought through a bit further. "You know the exercise has an awful lot to do with it. You could diet all day long and if you don't do some kind of exercise, you're dead. I don't care how good you are."

"Yes," says Bea, who has yet one more thing to say. "It's really terrific. I know that, because of living this life-style, my body is not the body of a fifty-four-year-old woman."

Comfortable in his chair, Alan doesn't respond to his wife's remark, but grins widely as she repeats it. "Yes, the Pritikin Program is terrific," Bea says emphatically. "The body is firm."

Chapter 2

Col. James B. Irwin, retired NASA astronaut; founder and now president of the High Flight Foundation, Colorado Springs, Colorado. Married with five children—one an adopted child from Vietnam.

Two heart attacks, plus bypass surgery.

Diagnosis: coronary artery disease.

Prognosis: poor.

I

"It was a shock to me. I thought, 'Man, Jim Irwin had a heart attack.' Someone who's as physically fit as I am. I have always been a physical fitness nut . . . I prided myself so much on being strong and healthy."

In the first moments of our conversation at the Colorado Springs office of the High Flight Foundation he now directs, astronaut Col. James B. Irwin summarized the effects of changing his life-style:

"It's been on my heart for several years to write a book about my experiences with the Pritikin Program. Not only did I regain the quality of my life and probably extend my life, but I can now do things that I thought were finished—like skiing and climbing mountains. And I can now do them with much more zest, much more energy than I ever did, even when I was a young man. I think this should be expressed clearly to encourage those who are facing a similar situation in their own life. And for young people, who could maybe make a change *before* they are threatened with severe health problems."

It is paradoxical to think of the words astronaut and heart disease in the same sentence. And still, there it is—a man whom we think of as having undertaken the most rigorous physical training on earth; a man who spent the major part of his life influenced by the disciplined

48

routines of the military and with access, supposedly, to the best in medical care—a man struck down in the prime of life by a disease usually associated with dietary excess, lack of exercise and general disregard for one's health, the disease of overwrought businessmen and uptight corporate managers, of heavy smokers and drinkers; the disease of caffeine, butter, eggs and red meat. But not the disease of astronauts.

For better or worse, Jim Irwin's story blasts holes in much of the common wisdom. The Apollo astronauts, for example, did not necessarily follow a scientifically regulated exercise regimen. They were not the recipients of the most enlightened health information. And they lived—contrary to their smiling PR images—under a great deal of accumulated stress.

Stress in its purest sense, says the dictionary, is "forcibly exerted influence." On what? Easily on the physical mechanisms of the body, forces that tend to strain or deform. Well-said words, indeed, but how do they translate? Perhaps they are most readily understood in one word: pressure, or its partner, tension. Something pushing on you that you can feel. Pressure to succeed, pressure to do your best, to feel happy; pressure not to feel guilty. The pressure of millions of tax-payer dollars riding on your back. The pressure of participating in a grand experiment on one hand, yet grounded in the simple reality of home and family on the other. Always trying to seek balance and rarely making it. Maybe not really wanting to make it.

Both Jim Irwin and his wife, Mary, have written books about the effects of Jim's astronaut experiences. Both testify to the new faith that has come to each in their own lives—Jim through his space experiences, Mary through long search and struggle. Jim's heart problems are mentioned almost incidentally in these books, appearing only as episodes among others in a larger struggle for self-awareness. But Jim's efforts to combat heart disease—in the face of being totally unprepared for its onslaught—are provocative. His experiences shatter the myths. In the suffering of his illness, Jim Irwin's experiences illustrate the tentative cords from which hang many of our modern medical truths. How he chose to confront his disease presents a challenge to others.

The voyage of Apollo 15 was a high point in America's space program, the proclamation of a more ambitious age of space flight. Apollo 15 was the first major scientific mission undertaken on the moon's surface—three days exploring the surface of the moon in an area called Hadley Rille—the first to bring back impressive samples of moon rocks, including the Genesis rock, thought to hold vital clues to the moon's geological evolution. Outside the Lunar Excursion Module

(LEM) for eight hours at a time, the astronauts–moon explorers investigated the geography of the moon's surface, deployed experiments and photographed their experiences.

The skipper of the Apollo 15 command module was Maj. Alfred M. (Al) Worden; the two lunar explorers Col. David R. (Dave) Scott and Col. James B. (Jim) Irwin. In publicity photographs taken during training and after their return to earth, the members of the Apollo 15 crew appear to conform to our expectations of NASA astronauts. They are clean-shaven, physically fit, mature in thought yet young in body, with steady eyes and a ready smile. Their faces exhibit an air of expectancy, their brash naivete is occasionally overshadowed by a suggestion of calm over-confidence. Three typically American men, not eccentric but daring, motivated not by individual success but by glory for their country and its space program. Three carefully selected individuals trained at great expense, destined to belong to one of the most exclusive clubs in the world—those who have experienced space.

Jim Irwin rejoiced in those days. Applying three times, he was accepted by NASA in 1966, into an astronaut class of nineteen other hopefuls. Admission to the astronaut program meant fulfillment of a long-time dream for this deceptively simple man, whose life prior to the NASA assignment bore small relationship to the all-American image that would be projected for him and his fellow recruits. If you look closely at the publicity photos from that time, past the hoopla and the smiles and the uniforms, you might catch a glimpse of Jim Irwin's complexity—a man with a purpose, yes, conflicting motives, yes. A man who is not all he seems and yet is much more.

At one point in our Colorado Springs interview, I ask Jim if there was ever any anxiety about whether or not he would be assigned a moon mission. His response is immediate.

"Oh, yes," he says, "there really was. There was a lot of pressure. And a lot of competition, particularly in my case, because my backup was Jack Schmidt—Harrison Schmidt—who was a professional geologist. He had a Ph.D. from Harvard, and there was a lot of pressure from the scientific community for a scientist to go to the moon. To show the guys how it should really be done," Jim adds dryly. "There had been a lot of pressure during my training," he repeats, "that maybe they'd let Jack Schmidt take my place. That's why I was so happy when I finally did lift off the earth. It was just such a joy. It couldn't be changed. I was destined for a space flight. At that point, no one could change his mind and put someone else in."

Irwin pauses thoughtfully and then continues. "It was a very happy moment, almost the happiest moment of my life, when I lifted off from the earth. But you never know if you're going to make it, because so many things can interfere, so many things can happen . . . and then someone else will take your place. Right down to the last minute. The tension is only relieved as you start to go into space and realize that you now have a chance to make your space flight—to do the things you trained to do for so many years. You live with that tension. It keeps building as the pressures get greater and greater.''

Jim hesitates a moment, as if to allow his train of thought a chance for a foothold. "Apollo 15 was a good flight—except that it turned out that we dehydrated ourselves, lost electrolytes like potassium and chromium. This was because of some of the physical ordeal of being on the moon and the poor diet we had in flight—the space food isn't that nutritious. Then there was the work we did on the surface and the great heat.

"All of this meant," he explains further, "that when Dave and I left the surface of the moon and went back into orbit, we had already developed heart irregularities." He drops this observation absently, as if the fact is common knowledge. I ask if anyone had foreseen this complication.

"No," he answers easily, "they never realized we'd work so hard. We were the first ones to spend three days on the surface. The others had been there about half that time. We were there during the heat of the day, and we were also given a lot more work to do. The drill, for example—taking more samples, covering more of the surface. We put a lot more work into to it, and we lost a lot of perspiration, lost a lot of electrolytes. That was NASA's explanation—loss of electrolytes. It was interesting," he reflects, "that both Dave and I developed the irregular heartbeat at about the same time—just shortly after we got back into orbit. The doctors on the earth could see it and they were a little alarmed.

"We realized we were dehydrated," he recalls, "because we'd been working hard. I couldn't get any water. No food. We didn't have time." He pauses, remembers, "They did give us a little bag of water inside the suit, but I could never suck the fluid out of it for some reason. Dave did drink out of his bag of water so he had some, but he was also working a lot harder than I was."

Fatigued but exhilarated by their three days of moon exploration, neither Scott nor Irwin was alarmed by their heart problem. "I didn't recognize it," says Jim. "I knew I was tired for the first time on the flight, but I'd never had heart irregularities before, so I didn't suspect it. Dave and I didn't discuss it. NASA wanted somehow to get the information to us, but they were afraid to tell us in plain language, because they feared the world would overreact—the press would overreact. The doctors, however, wanted at least to get the message to us, so they told Deke Slayton [Houston Control] to talk to the crew and tell us we should take something." Jim laughs faintly, remembering the NASA transmission. "What he said was 'Why don't you guys take a sleeping pill?' I received the message and I thought Deke was kidding. 'Take a sleeping pill? Man, we're exhausted; we don't need anything to go to sleep.' So I just disregarded his instructions. I thought it was just a casual comment. They didn't say why." Irwin thinks a moment. "I don't think I even mentioned it to Dave. I just thought, 'Well it's a joke. We're exhausted.' "

At this point in their journey, the Apollo 15 crew still had a two-day orbit of the moon to complete, followed by a two-day trip back to earth, a total of five more days before they would arrive home. "I don't know how long we had the irregular heartbeat," Jim observes, "but maybe when we woke up the next morning it was gone."

Jim Irwin has a habit of moving the conversation forward by using summarizing words or phrases. He injects one at this point. "So we had had some heart problems and we didn't find out about them until we came back to the earth and they told us, 'You guys had some rather severe heart arrhythmias after you left the moon. What do you think about that?' I remember I asked, 'Well, why didn't you tell us what the problem was so we could have reacted properly and taken the medication?' And then they said, 'We were afraid there would be an overreaction that might jeopardize future flights.' "

Like many of the astronauts before him—and as Tom Wolfe has documented in *The Right Stuff*—Irwin began his flying career as a test pilot in the program at Edwards Air Force Base in California's Mojave Desert. He moved his wife and the first of their three daughters to Edwards in 1960 and went to work. Soon enough he had earned himself a reputation. ". . . they always knew when Jim Irwin took off, because I would go right straight up in the most vertical way, on an angle that was a hairline from stalling."

Today Jim Irwin lives in Colorado Springs and runs the small Christian foundation he calls High Flight. His suite of offices is decorated with space memorabilia, from reproductions of moon rocks to commemorative plaques from the Apollo 15 mission. Immersed in this atmosphere, it takes a while to realize that the Apollo flight took place almost fifteen years ago. Here in the High Flight office, dominated by a wall-sized black-and-white photograph of the moon, it seems like it happened yesterday.

On the High Flight walls also hang testaments to Jim's new mission—a beautifully hand-crafted crucifix made from pieces of Western rocks and minerals, and other vaguely religious paintings and prints. Jim's office is open to the main part of the suite, separated by only a partial glass partition. From here, he can stand behind his desk and review his mail, take phone calls and call out soft instructions to one of his secretaries. The arrangement has the effect of making the whole suite—anteroom included—part of Jim's personal office, freeing him from the confines of conventional office space. Only his personal secretary, Kathy, has an enclosed office at the opposite end of the small suite. In all, the decoration is stylish and sophisticated.

Irwin himself has changed from the glory days. He's thinner now, still muscular but in a wiry rather than pumped-up way. You notice it first in his face. Earlier photos show a man who is well-padded, with curves. He is now a man of sharp angles; the bones in his face stand out. You think of finely executed porcelain struts underneath a rugged skin. The muscles under his blue velour jumpsuit ripple like taut wire. He could be any age between forty and fifty. In fact, he's fifty-five.

This Monday morning—a cold and windy, overcast Colorado spring day—I have been lucky to catch Col. Irwin in town. These days he spends most of his time traveling, speaking about the revelations of his space experiences. I wait on the couch, staring at the moon's portrait directly in front of me, while my host tends to some business. Inviting me in, we talk briefly in his office behind his glass partition; the phone rings, a few calls are taken. It becomes obvious that this won't do, and so we move to a small room set up as a theater, with a 16mm projector at the rear and chairs arranged in rows for an audience. The walls of this room are also covered with space memorabilia. Rearranging some of the chairs, we settle in, Jim with a yellow pad and felt-tipped pen resting on his knees, to take notes for the health book he hopes to write someday.

I first wanted to know if he enjoyed being on the moon.

"Yes," he answers, without qualification. "I felt at home there, like I was meant to be there. I guess because I've loved the mountains of the earth, and here we were in a little valley surrounded by the high mountains of the moon, the Ampernine Mountains that towered above us about 15,000 feet. It was spectacular scenery. It was also the ultimate desert. I'd spent a lot of my Air Force career in Arizona and in the Mojave Desert in California, and I came to love the desert. My wife doesn't like it at all. If she did, we'd probably be living in Yuma, Arizona." (Mary Irwin's impressions of desert heat and dust are well described in her own book and they are not complimentary.)

I ask Jim if Wolfe's scenario was correct, about there being a logical progression from test pilot to astronaut. "Yes," he says, "being an astronaut was a chance at fame and fortune and I wanted a little fortune." He laughs briefly. "I don't know if the fame was that important at that point, but I think there was also the desire to keep going higher and faster. For a pilot that's a natural progression.

"You are never completely satisfied. If there is a plane that will fly higher and faster, you want to fly it. I thought that space flight was probably the ultimate flight; I couldn't imagine anything higher or faster than that. So once it became obvious that man *could* go into space, I wanted to do *that*—that was a goal for my life."

He recalls, with a distinct fondness for the memory, "It goes back even to when I was a young boy, a very young boy. I had the feeling that I was going to be able to go to the moon some day. I told my father and mother and the people who lived around us that I was going to go to the moon. I have no idea where that came from—because this was way, way before the days of space flight. When I told my mother, she said, 'Son, that's foolishness. Man will never be able to go to the moon. So just forget that right now. I want you to do something worthwhile with your life.'

"She obviously didn't understand the dream," Jim observes. "But I figured that if I couldn't fly into space, I'll try to fly airplanes. Flying has just always been very exciting to me. On my first ride in an airplane as a passenger, I decided, 'Man, this is great; I'd like to be a pilot.' I had a chance to do a little flying at the Naval Academy, and then in the Air Force. There they formally prepared me as a pilot, and it did become very exciting and very satisfying—to keep going, flying all different types of airplanes, going higher and faster.

"Finally I had a chance to become a test pilot out at Edwards, working on the top secret YF-12A, which set speed and altitude records for the United States. However, just when I thought I had it made, I was involved in a very serious aircraft accident that left me a little crippled."

In her book, *The Moon Is Not Enough*, Jim's wife remembers vividly the incident that her husband refers to as "leaving him a little crippled." She was notified of Jim's accident at eight o'clock on a Sunday morning by two men "with grim expressions" who told her only that Jim appeared to have broken his leg. Because her thought was of a car accident, she asked her uniformed escorts about the location of Jim's car. "In the airport parking lot," came the reply. Instantly Mary Irwin grasped the gravity of the situation. At the hospital, Mary's only contact with her husband was with a figure swathed in bandages from head to feet who, although unconscious, was straining at the straps that held him on the stretcher. Mary describes her sense of desperation as she watched Jim being airlifted to a nearby base hospital. "The question that kept pounding at my already throbbing brain," she says, "was what should I do next? . . . I needed Jim to tell me."

Perhaps even more illustrative are the words Mary uses to characterize the routine of their life at Edwards: "Jim, out of necessity, left hurriedly early each morning, was gone all day, came in for a hastily consumed dinner, rushed to his desk and studied until late." That type of pace was to continue, in various permutations, throughout the couple's life.

Although Irwin says he "sustained" a long recovery period after the accident, there was actually some question as to whether he would ever walk again in a normal way. Most devastating, the doctors suspected he would never fly again, primarily because of severe head injuries. The matter-of-fact way Jim describes his accident prompts me to ask if there are many accidents testing planes.

"Yes," he responds. "A lot of men are killed testing airplanes. Flying an airplane is more dangerous than flying a spacecraft. But my accident wasn't even in a tester; it was just a little light airplane I was flying with a student."

Jim Irwin is not the child of a long-lined military dynasty, nor did he necessarily come to his military career out of patriotism or a sense of duty. Irwin's father was employed by the civil service, and his assignments gave the Irwin family the opportunity to travel to various parts of the country. "We were actually in Florida when the war started," Jim remembers. "We were there for a few years and then we moved west. After I left high school and went to the Naval Academy, my folks moved to California. My father died several years ago—the result of an accident. My mother's still alive. I was born in Pennsylvania and I lived in Florida and then Oregon for a very short period of time, and Utah, where I finished high school." He adds an important afterthought. "I've always been very physical," he says, "even though when I was in high school, I didn't have much time to participate in athletics."

Irwin's decision to enter the Naval Academy was primarily a matter of expediency. "I knew about the Naval Academy," he explains, "because I had visited there several times as a young man when we were living back East, and I was open to a military career. My father had served in the Army during the First World War, and he always said he was sorry he left it. So he encouraged me to consider a military career. I knew if I went to college, I'd have to work my way through—my folks couldn't provide the funds. So that meant a scholarship or an appointment to a military academy. In high school I tried to get a scholarship to Stanford, because I knew that was a very good school. I had good grades and I thought I could qualify, but I was turned down. My first thought then was to try to get an appointment to the military academy at West Point. Although they also turned me down, I was notified that I could get an alternative appointment to the Naval Academy. I decided I'd better take that because it was the only thing left. It turned out to be very good in the long run, although, while I was there, I didn't particularly enjoy it. There were many times when I wanted to resign.''

Jim Irwin's voice is soft and deep; it rolls around words like fine sandpaper smoothing off the edges of a rough board. It is free of harshness and barbs—the voice of a man who has spent much of his life expressing himself in front of others. He has a slight Southern accent, perhaps from his years in Houston, perhaps from his Southern experiences as a child. It is less a twang than a tendency toward unconventional accents on words. When he speaks of West Point, for example, the emphasis is on West, so it comes out *"West* Point.''

Irwin continues to detail his military career. "I was never a very military person, so I always kind of resented people trying to tell me what to do all the time. I knew that was necessary,'' he concedes, "but I didn't particularly like it. My folks encouraged me to go ahead and graduate from the Naval Academy, and I'm glad I stuck it out. And then, I guess probably I would never have continued with a military career if I hadn't decided I like to fly airplanes so much. That was something that seemed to be very satisfying.''

For Mary Irwin, there was never a time when Jim wasn't flying. Their courtship was sustained by Jim's weekend trips from Wright-Patterson Air Force base in Ohio, where he was stationed, to San Jose, California, where Mary lived. Jim had devised a system of shuttling personnel to the West Coast on weekends, thereby allowing him time to spend with Mary.

"As I flew,'' he says, "I continued to keep myself physically fit, or so I thought. I did bodybuilding all the way through my military career, even in the astronaut program. I ran a little bit. At the Naval Academy I ran cross-country at the intramural level and I was also on the track team for a while, but I really didn't enjoy running. When I got into the astronaut program, some of the people were running, and I thought maybe it would be a nice thing to do. So I'd run, maybe a mile at the most, never really doing an extended distance.''

Although it might seem that cardiovascular fitness would be an important aspect of military training, Jim's experiences indicate this is not true. "At the Naval Academy," he recollects, "I was really big on bodybuilding; I built up big muscles during that time. But it really wasn't encouraged that much. That's something I took on. You see," he continues, "when you first enter the academy, they assign an upper-classman to kind of be your mentor or counselor. Actually mine se-lected me. He was a tremendously strong man from New Mexico, and he was big into bodybuilding. He had built up tremendously large muscles. I guess the first time I saw him he impressed me because he was walking up to his room on his hands. He could even climb stairs on his hands. He impressed me, and so I tried to pattern my life after him in many ways while I was at the Naval Academy. I lifted weights, but I also did some gymnastics, played squash, did some running. My big emphasis, however, was building muscles, particularly in my upper body. I was rather skinny—light—when I left high school and I was a little embarrassed at the way I looked, so this was an opportunity for me."

Ironically the type of bodybuilding Irwin pursued throughout most of his military career and even into retirement, while helping to define muscles, actually works contrary to cardiovascular conditioning. Lifting weights can cause a rise in blood pressure, and place a strain on the heart. Jim further complicated his potential health problems by enjoying unabashedly the substantial food available to him as a cadet.

"I guess that's also why I ate so much of that rich food," he says, "because I thought, 'Well, that will help me in my bodybuilding.' Because of what's happened since then, I realize that the heart is really the most important muscle in the body, and if you're going to emphasize any particular muscle, it should be the heart. I learned a lot, but it took me a long while to get there. At the time, I just figured I could work off any excess fat that I was taking in. At the academy, the diet was very rich food that I had really not had much of before because my folks were—I won't say poor, that's probably not the right word to use—probably of modest income. We always had enough to eat but we didn't have an abundance of food, and what we had was prepared in a simple fashion. We lived a rather simple life-style. For many years, we didn't even have an automobile.

"Then I went off to the Naval Academy and there was butter and milk in abundance, and meat. So, man, I ate a lot. I put on about thirty pounds, I'd guess. It was mostly muscle, but there was also probably a lot of fat. When I was at home, I don't think we ever had butter. But at the academy there was butter and I just got carried away with it. We'd literally use sticks of it; we put it on bread just really thick, not realizing the effect that it would have later on in life. And then milk, rich milk from the dairy there at the Naval Academy. When we had ice cream at home, it was a real treat, but at the Naval Academy we had dessert at each meal. I thought it was great. I was a young man, very active athletically, so I thought I could certainly burn off any fat I might be gaining. And I kept building and building up muscles that would never really benefit me—other than to build up my ego, I guess—so I'd look good, look strong. I think I began the trend that led to my heart problems many years later.

"And after graduation," he continues, "when I went into the military, I was making fairly good money. I got married and my wife always fixed good food, not overly rich but the typical American diet. As we moved up the ladder, we ate richer and richer. And after becoming an astronaut—particularly after a flight to the moon, everybody wants to feed you the richest, the very best food—or so-called best food—wherever you travel. I think that eating like that contributed to my downfall. I admit that I enjoyed the food, and certainly I ate my share," he laughs. "And probably someone else's share."

"I sometimes wonder," he suggests, "if when you come from a rather poor background where you don't have enough to eat, maybe when you do or you can afford it, you subconsciously try to make up for those years you were hungry. I know that's very obvious in the case of our adopted son from Vietnam. He must have had some years when he was really starving because now he just stuffs himself."

Things haven't changed much at the Naval Academy since Jim Irwin graduated. A recent review of the food served naval cadets (in none other than *Gourmet* magazine) seems to indicate that the Navy has turned a deaf ear to recent concern about dietary fat and cholesterol. Milk and ice cream—some 300 gallons a day—still come from the academy's herd of dairy cows. Containers of milk are placed on every table in the mess hall at every meal, along with a jar each of crunchy and smooth peanut butter—no cholesterol but lots of fat. Food service statistics are the most revealing. On an average day, the kitchen will serve 1,000 gallons of whole milk, 1,200 loaves of bread, two tons of meat, another two of potatoes, one ton of green vegetables, 720 pies and all those gallons of ice cream. The kitchen can turn out 3,000 hamburgers and a ton of French fries in an hour. The Navy makes its own doughnuts in the academy bakery and serves them for breakfast along with cereal, oatmeal, eggs, bacon, sausage, potatoes, bagels and cream cheese, coffee and hot chocolate. Common entrées include roast beef, cold cuts, Wiener schnitzel, "surf and turf," barbecued spareribs and fried shrimp. "The Navy stresses food," says Lieutenant Commander Doug Peart, the Midshipman Food Officer at the academy. "Always has."

I wondered how astronaut training differed from Irwin's experiences at the Naval Academy. "It was pretty busy," Jim remembers. "We were busy all the time: flying airplanes and helicopters, flying simulators, running geological field trips all around the world; traveling a good deal. Trying to learn all we thought was necessary to do the flight. In five years we'd completed all the training. There was always the prime crew and the back-up crew; there were six of us who went through almost the same kind of training. And there were also crews training for other flights. I guess at any one time, there might have been from fifteen to twenty of us training for a moon flight."

Irwin describes the training atmosphere as competitive. "There was a certain comradery" he explains, "but each group of astronauts was on its own. We knew that the ones selected a year or two before us would be the commanders and we would be going as their helpers. There were nineteen men selected when I was and after about a year of training together, they farmed us out for various jobs such as learning a specific procedure or piece of equipment. I was given the assignment of monitoring the development of the lunar module and performing some of the testing on the space suit. For me, it was a lucky break. I had always figured, 'If I fly in space—and particularly if I fly to the moon—I don't want to just *circle* the moon, I want to go down and *land* on it.' And so because of the training work, I became recognized as an expert on the lunar module. That made it easier for me to qualify eventually for the flight.

"After training, I worked on the support crew for Apollo 10 and back-up crew for Apollo 12 and finally, my big chance on Apollo 15." He totals up the experience. "That meant," he says, "I worked as back-up and prime crew on a lunar mission for a total of three years. The last three, we worked together as a team." These are comfortable memories, easily resurrected. He recalls, "We worked very hard. Each day was very full from the beginning, and we worked right through into the evening. The last six months before our flight, we lived down at the Kennedy Space Center and went home only on weekends. The family," he remembers, "was living in Houston at that point."

It was during Jim's Houston training that Mary Irwin experienced full-force what it meant being married to an ambitious and extremely self-motivated individual. After a brief nine months in Colorado Springs—a climate and atmosphere she loved—Mary and her four children were re-routed to Houston. Everything about Houston bothered

Mary—the endless flat Texas landscape, the dismal muddy cast of shallow Galveston Bay, the small apartment Jim had selected as their temporary quarters. Worst of all was the formidable pressure of her husband's commitment to NASA's schedule. Mary describes vividly in her book how she finally "cracked":

"One summer morning while the children were outside playing, I washed and set my hair and began cleaning the house. While absent-mindedly pushing the vacuum about the living room, my mind seemed weighted as I brooded over what seemed a hopeless set of circumstances. Tears of self-pity started to flow. I switched off the vacuum, sat down on the sofa, and mulled over events of the past few months. Our problems loomed insurmountable in my mind, and I became inwardly frustrated, fatigued. Wearily I lay down on the sofa . . . and staring emptily into space, I slipped into a mental trance. As I lay there, I gave up hope and totally withdrew from my surroundings."

Mary spent a brief period in the psychiatric ward of a local hospital, but her near-breakdown did little to alleviate the problems that plagued her and her family. Jim remained committed to his dream of space flight, receiving satisfaction from his training challenges, but Mary, unable to reconcile Jim's motivated vision with the realities of her own family's life, found it difficult to build inner strength or self-esteem. Before she met and married Jim Irwin, Mary Monroe had embarked on what promised to be a successful modeling career. She surrendered that goal when she married Jim, substituting the values of home and family for the rewards of a career. Although she never mentions regret at that choice, her words are full of frustration at Jim's and her inability to develop a "normal" family life against the backdrop of his military career.

Considering that Mary's words are so much more impassioned than Jim's cooler description of that time, I asked Jim if it had been difficult to be involved in a program so intensely. His answer comes easily. "No," he says, "because we knew this was the chance of a lifetime, that if we really were fortunate, we'd get a chance to fly in space. So I gave myself to it wholeheartedly. I thought it was the most important thing I could do with my life at that point. We were all dedicated and we wanted to fly in space in the worst way, whatever it took, even if it meant the sacrifice of our relationships with our families. And many did," he admits. "I think I was guilty of that too. We worked extremely hard, but we never looked at it like that; we figured this was what was required to go into space."

Irwin notes that during astronaut training there was little of the superfluous military drilling that had irritated him at the Naval Academy. "We knew that all of what we were doing was necessary," he says. "Everything was done in a practical way—'This is what you must learn; this is how you must operate; this is how you have to act if you're going to be successful in space.' Everything was geared to that goal, and we had a significant input. We'd question things, and if we didn't get the correct answer, we changed them. We were all learning a lot about the space environment, the space hardware and a lot about ourselves as we prepared for the flight. We were learning to adjust to living with two other people for a long period of time in a small space craft. And," he adds significantly, "learning to live in a suit."

When I appear perplexed by that statement, he explains, "Living in a space suit can be a real experience; you can get claustrophobic. I just wondered how I could possibly live in that suit for days at a time. Gradually you come to accept it, but it's still difficult. Just recently I had a space suit on in Dallas for a special program. I didn't even have the helmet on, but I thought, 'Phew, how did I live this way for so many years?' "

Irwin credits his eventual acceptance as an astronaut to his persistence and commitment to his dream of space. "On my third application," he admits, "I didn't hold too much hope because they'd turned me down twice before. I was at the age limit and I wasn't even a test pilot anymore. I had a desk job. But there were some senior officers here at Colorado Springs, as well as at headquarters, who really went to bat for me, were convinced of my potential and believed that I should have a chance."

As far as any repercussions from his crash at Edwards, Irwin says he made "a complete recovery," and although he considers it "amazing," he was back on flight status about two years after the accident. "I think," he reflects, "that the serious head injuries, the concussion, the loss of memory did not make me a very suitable candidate to become an astronaut. I'm sure that's why they turned me down when I tried the first time. The second time they were just looking for people with a doctoral degree. I didn't have one."

Although Jim glosses over the extent of the accident, Mary Irwin provides a more detailed description of his injuries and his long period of recuperation. She recalls that their oldest daughter, Joy, was so frightened by her father's bandaged appearance—after not having seen him for months during his recuperation—that she ran from his arms and remained aloof for some time. Jim's seemingly blasé attitude about what would appear to have been a major set-back in his dream of flying ever higher and faster repeats itself in other incidents throughout his life. The image emerges of a man who attacks challenges full-force, takes the repercussions in the same spirit and then commits prodigious energy and determination to righting adverse circumstances.

But Irwin is a man capable of considerable insight about his experiences. When asked of his thoughts upon his return from the moon, he answered, "When you come back from a space flight, you don't feel very normal. You just feel completely drained. There's literally a physical change that takes place during a space flight. Even if you're up there for just a week, there's a change. We were up there for twelve days, and it took us almost three weeks before we satisfied the doctors and the medical community that we were almost normal.

"The changes that take place are well documented," he explains. "You change physically, psychologically and even spiritually. You lose weight, you lose body fluids—the body realizes that you don't need all those fluids and starts casting them off. You lose red blood cells, and because you don't need strong bones in space, calcium production begins to decrease. And there's a "deconditioning" of the cardiovascular system because the heart can do its function—distribute blood around the body—without gravity. The head begins to swell and the sinuses are clogged because of the pressure. There's also more blood in the extremities."

Strange as it may appear, the astronauts were not provided a specific reconditioning program on their return from the moon. Jim recalls they simply went back to their pre-flight routine. "And it wasn't long," he says, "before the doctors said we were normal, almost normal—playing handball or racquetball or lifting weights or swimming. We were always very active, both before and after the flight." He pauses and then says thinly, "I don't think you're ever completely normal, however." There is another pause before he expands on his statement. "I'm talking about the psychological effect of space flight.

"Psychologically," he explains, "I think who we are is the result of how we think others perceive us. That's how we form our self-esteem and our self-image. So after your first space flight, everybody regards you as somehow different, even your closest friends. You're never really the same." He hesitates, thinking through his supposition carefully. "Even within a close, intimate group of friends, friends you've known most of your life, someone will inevitably introduce you to a new person with, 'Oh, meet my friend Jim; he's been to the moon.'

"And so it's not the Jim Irwin he or she knew before; it's the Jim Irwin who's *been to the moon*. Somehow that Jim Irwin's not the same anymore. He's different because he's been to a different place, a place to which they'll probably never go. So for you life takes on a new meaning. You're different in their eyes, and thus you're different, I think, in your own eyes.''

Without prompting he begins to describe his own personal changes. ''I was different for many reasons. Because of everything that happened to me, I came back with a new perspective, a new appreciation for earth, a new appreciation for life, a new love for the people on the earth. Life became much, much fuller and richer as a result of the flight.''

Although continually busy during the moon mission, Jim reflects, ''What really got our attention most and what was the most lasting was the earth—seeing it so beautiful. Small enough that you could hold it in your hands and eventually small enough so you could hold it between your fingers. And realizing, 'Man, that's my home and everything I can relate to is out there, but it's in miniature.' You come back with a great perspective about how small it is and yet how significant it is.''

Recrossing his legs and resettling himself in the chair, he continues to elaborate. ''And things took place on the surface of the moon that had great impact for me, great spiritual meaning—like finding the Genesis Rock, the only white rock returned from the moon. There were prayers that were answered just immediately when we were working on the moon's surface. And inspiration to quote scripture, which I'd never done before. It just seemed like the Lord had been part of the mission, had been with me and now wanted to use me in a different way. He'd given me a flight to the moon, but now he wanted me to share that flight, wanted me to share his message really, with the people of the earth—to make all of us appreciate the Blue Planet more. To appreciate one another; love each other more.''

Irwin is not alone in his reactions to his space experiences. ''We all came back,'' he says, ''with that distinct impression and the desire to share that feeling, and many of us are very active doing that. It's something we have in common.'' He emphasizes the words something and do, implying the continued bond. ''We've all tried to somehow project that to the people on the earth so that they might feel what we've felt. Because, you know, we were only able to do that because we had the support of thousands, millions of people. We're trying to give them back something they paid for. After all,'' he muses in conclusion, ''our trip to the moon was one of man's great adventures.''

II

"We had our own chef. He'd been a chef on a yacht . . . he was great at fixing cakes and pies and steaks."

Jim's secretary, Kathy Duncan, has interrupted us with telephone messages that require attention. Jim directs me across the hall for a cup of herb tea from the snack bar. As the day has progressed, the temperature seems to have dropped in the face of a stiff wind and a reluctant sun. I streak back across the open courtyard to the warmth of the High Flight office, my tea quietly splashing from side to side in the plastic cup. Jim and I take our respective seats, he rotating one of the extra chairs to use as an armrest.

The astronaut's story continues:

"In 1973 I was down in Houston for my annual check-up; NASA still encourages us to go down there on a yearly basis to see if there are any long-term effects from our space experience. They said then, 'You're in great shape. No problems. The stress test was successful again.'

"I had retired from the space program by then and although I knew that I wasn't feeling quite as good as I had the year before, I came back from Houston and was busier than ever." He stops, says noncommittally, "I was working harder after I retired than I had been before. At that time I had three jobs. I was trying to head up this foundation. I was doing consulting work at Johns-Manville Corporation in Denver, and I was also doing some radio and broadcasting work with the Radio and Television Commission of the Southern Baptist Convention in Fort Worth. And I was also flying myself around the country to most of my engagements. I was doing so much flying, in fact, that I thought I was justified in getting a Lear jet.

"So at about that time, I was in the process of qualifying for a license. I wasn't aware of it then, but the day I was scheduled to take the written test, I probably set myself up for what was to come." He adjusts the chair he's using as an armrest so it's more comfortable. "I overslept," he says, "which got me off to a bad start. I had to drive to Denver to take the exam." (The route from Colorado Springs to Denver is about 100 miles, mostly four-lane highway, and much of it through relatively deserted country.) "There'd been a snowstorm the night before," he continues, "and there was a lot of snow and ice on the road. I took off, with no breakfast, in my little car, and about two miles outside of the ranch, I slid off the road. I had to hitchhike back into town to get a tow truck to pull me out of the ditch. Finally I got back on the road and had to really whip to Denver in order to make the examination.

"I made it," he says flatly, "and I worked through the exam, but I didn't have time for lunch because I knew I was scheduled to play handball at about two o'clock.

"So," he summarizes, "here I am concentrating on this examination, which was really tough. I'd had no food and had gone right from the examination over to the gym to play handball. I was just beginning to warm up with the guys, hitting the ball, when suddenly I felt nauseated. I felt pressure in my chest, like I couldn't breathe. There was also some pain in my arms. So I asked the guys if they'd excuse me and I went into a rest room there. I figured with just a little relaxation I'd feel OK."

I asked Jim if he could describe the difference in his physical health between 1973 and the previous year. "I think the thing that bothered me the most," he says thoughtfully, "was that I didn't have time for exercise. Before—I guess all the time I was in the military and with NASA—physical fitness had been a priority, and I was always able to schedule it. But when I was retired and on my own, there were many days when I'd go without exercise at all, and it was difficult. It bothered me that I wasn't getting the exercise I thought I should have. And physically you miss it; you get real tight. I was playing handball and lifting weights, but not running—that wasn't something I enjoyed. And I noticed I was putting on weight. That was difficult to handle."

Mindful that the long-term Framingham study of heart disease has reported that men and woman twenty percent or more above the median weight for their age and sex have twice the risk of developing heart disease than those below it, I asked Jim if he would describe himself as severely overweight or just heavier than usual. "I was heavier than I wanted to be," he answers. "My clothes were getting a little tight. I knew I was heavier, but I always figured if someone's going to have a heart attack, it's going to be someone who's really overweight, who drinks, smokes, and who just isn't taking care of himself."

According to his NASA records, which plot not only his health profile but those of the entire astronaut group, Irwin's weight didn't change dramatically either during astronaut training or after the space flight, although the excess pounds he felt may have been the transformation of once tightly toned muscle into fat. His cholesterol, however, did show a sharp rise, especially compared to the rest of the astronaut group. In 1966, for example, when he entered the program, Irwin's cholesterol was just below 260; it dropped briefly during training, hitting a low of 200 in 1970, only to jump to 260 in 1971, the year of Apollo 15. From there it continued a steady rise to 320 in 1976, a time when, although he was experiencing heart difficulties, he continued to pursue his extraordinarily demanding lifestyle. In 1973, the year he's speaking of here, his blood cholesterol was 300. During his NASA years and after, Irwin's blood pressure fluctuated considerably, hitting highs in 1972 and 1973 just after the moon flight and again in 1977 and '76, coinciding with his high cholesterol levels.

Had anyone taken the time to monitor these values with any thought to their long and short-term implications, Jim might have had sufficient warning of what lay ahead. Instead he found himself in the men's room on a Colorado Air Force base, nauseous and suffering from unfamiliar pain. "I was in the restroom and I vomited," he remembers, "but I hadn't had anything to eat. I figured something was really wrong with me and I had the presence of mind to call the base hospital and have them send over an ambulance. At that point," he discloses, "I didn't have any fear of a heart attack. You see, I had never had any angina—any chest pains. I just thought, 'This feeling is going to pass and I'll be able to play handball.'

"Well anyway," he summarizes thinly, dismissing his previous observation, "they picked me up and took me over to the base hospital. The doctor who met me at the door recognized the symptoms. He said, 'We're not even going to try to treat you here; we'll send you over to Fitzsimons,'—the Army medical center—which was close by. He didn't say what was wrong—at least I don't think he did. They had me in the emergency room and within thirty minutes started treating me for heart attack. After that they took me to intensive care. I was in the hospital, I guess, for three weeks. When I was released, I began a gradual rehabilitation program."

For independent, strong-willed Jim Irwin, to be struck down by a heart attack at forty-three, in what he thought of as "the prime of my life," was quite a blow. "I always figured," he concedes, "that if I could go to the moon, I could do anything, and here I'd had a heart attack. It was a great shock," he repeats. "It really hung over me. I realized I was just as weak as others; in fact, I was in worse shape than most. Here were overweight people who had never had a heart attack, and here I was, supposedly a physical specimen . . . I was really the first astronaut to have a heart attack," he concludes.

I asked him what NASA thought. "Well," he begins, "it turned out, looking at my medical record, that my cholesterol had continued to rise over the years. But they hadn't clearly pointed that out. No one had told me that it was gradually going up. They said after it was over,

'Didn't we tell you that the cholesterol was going up?' I said, 'No.' Maybe they had,'' he speculates, ''maybe I just passed over it.

"I never really smoked, just a little bit when I was a young fighter pilot or cigars when someone had a baby. And I always thought I was eating fairly healthy. Steak was still a desirable meal for me, however, and I'd probably have dessert too, cake or pie or ice cream. They didn't have a very good rehabilitation program at Fitzsimons at that time, and when I went back to the ranch, my instructions were to cut down on cholesterol, reduce it if I could, although they didn't really tell me how to do it. And they said, 'When you feel your strength come back, get some exercise. Start walking.' But when I got home," recalls Jim wearily, "I just collapsed into bed—it was so good to be home. It was a while before I started walking, but I did eventually. It was a very slow rehabilitation."

I asked Jim what Mary thought about the heart attack. "She was probably just as shocked as I was," he says, "but I think she realized I was probably trying to do too much anyway, that something would happen to me, that some sort of an exhaustion was bound to set in." Irwin coughs up a little self-mocking laughter here, as if he might, too, have come to the same realization, but was too busy to do anything about it. "I was aware," he grants, "that I was trying to do too many things, plus flying myself around the country. There were times when I was flying that I would wonder, 'Am I flying to the right place today?' " He laughs again, this time unfolding a kind of engaging smile. "Sometimes I did land at the wrong airport." I laugh with him at the image created by his words: a former astronaut, used to the rarified atmosphere of space, lost in the closer skies above home territory.

"Do you consider yourself a Type A?" I asked.

Irwin nods his head yes but doesn't elaborate. He chooses instead to proceed with his story by way of describing the first of his efforts to discover a program to aid in his rehabilitation and protect himself against further heart attacks. In 1973 on a trip to Los Angeles, he met a well-known nutritionist who claimed that Jim suffered from hypoglycemia. To relieve the problem, Jim's newfound counselor prescribed a high protein diet supplemented with mega-vitamins and lecithin. Eating the cheese, red meat and milk prescribed for his erroneously diagnosed low blood sugar, Irwin's heart condition continued to deteriorate as his cholesterol rose.

Jim easily admits he was depressed during that time. "There were so many things I wanted to do. That was the year I was supposed to go to Ireland," he recalls. "I'd always wanted to go back to Ireland because my father was from Irish roots. I also thought that I should visit Ireland in my new mission. I was invited to dedicate the new YMCA in Belfast. That very month, in the spring of '73, I had the heart attack, so I had to cancel. I had engagements scheduled for years ahead of time, and I had to cancel a lot of them. This bothered me," he says, "because I always try to keep my commitments."

During the summer after Jim's attack, the High Flight Foundation had scheduled a spiritual retreat for former prisoners of war and those who had been "missing in action" in Vietnam. Some 1,500 people had been invited. Irwin, just recovering from his heart problems, consulted his physician on the advisability of a visit to the retreat's mountain site. His doctor suggested that he confine his trip to a few days. Stubborn and used to defying the odds, however, Irwin visited the retreat; he enjoyed it so much, felt so comfortable and got so involved with the participants that he stayed for the duration, which meant he spent the entire summer at an altitude of almost 8,000 feet. And this only months after he had a major heart attack.

Jim characterizes his recovery as slow, because "I wasn't following any change in diet. And I wasn't really pushing myself as far as exercise. In about six months—the fall of that year—I was back to my normal speaking and traveling schedule. But I knew then that I just didn't have the mental resources or physical energy to continue with my other two jobs. So I just devoted myself to High Flight. I wasn't flying myself anymore, either. I knew I wanted to fly, but it took about a year to get my medical clearance back.

"So there I was," he recaps, "taking all these vitamins and getting busy again but not feeling very well. Then, in the fall of 1977, four years later, one of my friends here invited me to play handball with him. I hadn't played much handball since I had the heart attack. I'd also missed lunch the day we were going to play so I grabbed some cheese to eat beforehand. I got on the court and I started playing and then began burping up the cheese.

"I just brushed it off, thinking, 'Well it's because I've eaten too much cheese for my hypoglycemia.' But I really just felt horrible, and I knew that something wasn't right. So the next day I went up to the Air Force Academy and asked them for a stress test. Well, I got on the treadmill, and it wasn't long before the doctor said, 'Yes, you've got a problem; better get off.' "

Typically, a stress test for heart patients provides an indication of their heart rate, as well as evidence of any damage or recovery from damage caused by previous attacks or coronary incidents. The test is completed on a computerized treadmill, with controlled variations in speed and resistance (achieved by adjusting the treadmill's slope). As the patient walks through his paces, a physician and/or technician monitors the electrocardiogram reading, which provides an indication of the contractions of the heart muscle under the various degrees of workload controlled by the treadmill. While the output of an electrocardiogram may show no abnormalities in a person's heart at rest, loading the heart and forcing an increased demand for oxygen—the premise of the stress test—is likely to cause reactions if the individual's coronary arteries are blocked and his heart is not receiving a sufficient supply of oxygen-carrying blood.

Jim's Air Force doctors were "so convinced" he had blockage from atherosclerosis plaques in his coronary arteries that they advised a trip to the Veterans Administration Hospital in Denver for an angiogram and probable bypass surgery.

"As soon as I heard that," says Jim, "I called NASA and told them what was in the wind. They responded, 'If there's any possibility that you're going to need that, we'd like you to come down to Houston because we'd like you to have the very best treatment. We'd like Denton Cooley to check you out.' "

NASA's preference for Denton Cooley is understandable. In a field dominated by superstars, Dr. Cooley is a legend in his own time. Located at the Texas Heart Institute, formerly a partner with another bypass hero, Michael DeBakey, Cooley is considered one of the men to see when coronary bypass surgery is indicated.

Astronaut Irwin decided to take NASA's advice and visit Houston for the angiogram and possible surgery. "I made arrangements, I think, in about a week or two, to go down to Houston," he remembers. "Cooley looked at the results of the angiogram and agreed that there was blockage in the coronary arteries, which he put at seventy and fifty percent."

It is generally considered that a coronary artery that is blocked *up to* seventy percent of its normal capacity due to plaque buildup will, in most cases, not produce symptoms of pain or discomfort except under stress—physical or emotional. If blockage increases past seventy to eighty percent, however, even small changes in the heart's workload can produce the severe pain of angina. An artery that is ninety percent blocked may result in angina symptoms even at rest. So it's conceivable that even with his blockage, Jim might have felt no symptoms until he exposed his heart to an accelerated workload—such as a handball game— or a stress test. It is conceivable also, that a highly motivated—and sometimes self-deceiving—person like Jim could quite simply *ignore* angina symptoms.

Jim relates that Cooley assessed that the blockage in his arteries was "significant" and recommended he have bypass surgery. Says Irwin, "At that time—January 1977—I wasn't aware of any alternative treatment so I had Cooley perform the bypass."

I asked if the need for surgery caused any further concern about how he had developed a heart condition in the first place. Jim ponders that for a long moment and says, "No-o-o, not yet."

"No anger?" I asked.

"No," he answers. "Not yet."

Col. Irwin experienced a good recovery from his triple bypass and went back to Colorado Springs to work with the cardiologist who had originally administered the stress test at the Air Force Academy. He claims he recovered "very quickly," and since it was a good year for skiing, he requested, in late March, permission from his doctor to accompany his family on a trip to Vail. His physician, however, passed the ball back into the Irwin court, advising Jim that it depended on how he felt, how his chest felt (there is usually considerable chest pain after bypass surgery) and Irwin's own assessment of his energy level.

Jim admits, "This was two months after the surgery and I realized I was pushing it. But I went skiing anyway." Then with a tight expulsion of breath, he says, "And riding up on the chair lift, I had a second heart attack, right there on the lift."

It's difficult to imagine more inhospitable circumstances for someone with a heart condition—high altitude, frigid air, relative inaccessibility to immediate medical aid. "I was fortunate," he says distantly, "to have our youngest daughter with me, because I was nauseous. I felt like I was going to fall off the chair. She held on to me until we got to the top. But it was so cold there that I didn't want to just wait for the ski patrol to bring oxygen to me and take me down. So I said to my daughter, 'Let's ski down the mountain.' " He adds, "I had to stop on the way down several times."

I asked if he knew what was happening to him. "I knew it was a heart attack," he says. "I told my daughter what was happening, and she was really frightened. She was probably about twelve or thirteen, but she stayed right with me and managed to get me down to midmountain. I decided maybe I should wait there. I went into the building, stretched out on the floor and waited for them to bring the oxygen to me. It seemed like it took forever. Finally they got the oxygen and they took me down on a sled, on a toboggan, to the bottom of the mountain. My wife was there with the car. I got into the car, and I said, 'Just take me back to the place where we're staying. I'll be all right in a day or two.' But Mary realized there was something really wrong," he continues, "that I was really having a problem. I was not in pain but I was very uncomfortable."

"A feeling of suffocation?" I asked.

"Suffocation, yes," he answers, then he stops, and after a long pause, says, "I did feel nauseated like I was the first time and I had a strong suspicion it was a heart attack, very strong. Mary insisted I go over to the Vail medical center, and they confirmed that I had had another heart attack. For three days they tried to stabilize my condition. My heart rate was very erratic, my blood pressure . . . Finally in desperation as it were, they said, 'We're going to have to call the Army and airlift you out of here.' Well, fortunately the Army sent a helicopter up to Vail that took me and Mary down to Fitzsimons. As soon as we got down to a lower altitude, I felt much better. Vail, you see, is about 9,000 feet. So," he concludes with a humorless chuckle, "there I was back in Fitzsimons—where I'd started.

"And again three weeks in the hospital. This time they had a very good rehabilitation program; strict low-cholesterol diet and exercise, mostly walking. I enjoyed it. Later—it was during the summer—someone sent me a copy of Nathan's first book." Jim is speaking slowly now, assembling events and anecdotes. ". . . *Live Longer Now*. I read it. It really made sense to me, and then I realized all the foolishness I'd listened to—you know, the mistakes."

I asked Jim if after all of this, the attacks and the bypass, he had begun to experience any anger at NASA.

"No," he responds at first, "I wasn't . . ." Then he admits, "Well, I was somewhat angry at NASA—because they were never big on health food. We could eat anything we wanted. Because we were living in our crew quarters at the Kennedy Space Center, we had our own chef. He'd been a chef on a yacht and didn't appear to know anything about nutrition. He would just say, 'Hey, you guys just tell me what you'd like to eat and I'll fix it for you.' He was great at making cakes and pies and fixing steaks. No one seemed to be monitoring the astronauts' diet.

"Before the flight," Jim says, "we had a chance to taste the space food and decide what we liked . . . that helped determine what we should take into space. It was mostly freeze-dried, and provided only calories and the flavor; it wasn't that good nutritionally. The morning of the flight, they asked what we wanted for breakfast. We said, 'Well, we'll have steak and eggs and pancakes.' And we had a huge, huge breakfast. When we came back from the moon, what was the first thing we wanted? Steak and ice cream on the carrier. So obviously we weren't eating right. It was just like our physical program. They said,

'You guys are smart enough to know you should be in good condition. You just design your own program.' So we designed our own physical fitness program. And we ate the way we thought we should eat.

"That was it."

III

"Every day is a day of fresh commitment. It's like a sense of renewal."

Jim Irwin discovered the Pritikin Program through one of the Pritikin books that described the recommended diet and exercise program. "I read it and it really made sense," Jim says. Primed to be receptive at that point, Jim received additional support from a long-time friend.

"In the fall of '77 an old friend called me—Chick Stevens, who used to be a pilot for Frontier and is now involved in their in-flight magazine. Chick had just come back from the Pritikin center in Santa Barbara, where he'd gone because he'd had a stroke. He said to me, 'Jim, this is the program you should get on. It's made a big difference in my life.' So with Chick's strong insistence that I try it, I made it my New Year's resolution, that as of the first of January 1978, I would follow this program."

Jim maintains he "couldn't afford the time" or that $6,000 price tag, to participate in the program at the Pritikin center. Neither, however, stopped him from independently evaluating and revamping his life-style. As he struggled to implement the Pritikin approach, in the spring of 1978, another good friend contacted him, "out of the blue," as Jim explains it, and told him, "I'm going up to visit this Colorado Health Center where they have a program based on Nathan Pritikin's, and I'm going to pick you up and take you there with me today." Although surprised, Irwin agreed to make the trip. During the tour of the center, he met with the director and the center's staff and accepted their invitation to return for two weeks and participate in their program. He recalls, "As a result of doing that—I hadn't done any exercise up to that time—they had me walking again. In fact they got me jogging for the first time.

"I felt so good with the diet, which I'd started in January, and with the encouragement I received there at the center, that I improved quickly," he remembers enthusiastically. "I started jogging every day and I really liked it. I knew that I was getting stronger and the quality of life was coming back.''

Although Irwin doesn't describe how he was feeling previous to his visit to the center, the fact that he was enthused about renewed walking and jogging suggests his formerly active life-style had been radically curtailed.

Another important benefit of his stay at the Colorado Health Center was that Jim discontinued his medication, which included Norpace, a drug to help regulate his erratic heart beat; Persantine, a vasodilator; and aspirin, a blood thinner. An even bigger bonus, he remembers, was that by summer he was able to climb Pikes Peak for the first time in years. "From that point, I just kept getting better," he remembers. "I've been on the program now since 1978, and have more energy than I'd ever dreamed would be possible. Being able to ski again and ski much harder than I had before, skiing to the point where my kids wear out and I can continue. Being able to climb mountains. This was wonderful," he says emphatically, "because when I had the second heart attack, I was completely wiped out. I thought I'd never be able to do the things that I really liked to do.

"The first heart attack," he continues, "was a warning. I thought I would probably recover after the first one, but when the second one hit, then I wondered, you know, if something really very serious was going on. I thought," he says flatly, "I might not be here very long. So I'm indebted to Nathan for the fact that I'm still here, that life continues, that the quality of life is increased to the point that I can not only climb Pikes Peak but I can go over and climb Mt. Ararat in Turkey and look for Noah's Ark.''

Real joy warms Jim's voice as he concludes his testimony. "After my attacks, I never dreamed I'd be looking for Noah's Ark, never dreamed I'd be climbing Mt. Ararat. I thought things like that were finished. But to be able to climb to the top of a 17,000-foot mountain, to be able to do it as well as those who've never had a heart attack, is just amazing to me. So I know that the body can recover, that we have a marvelous healing mechanism. I think that I have a new heart, or new circulation to my heart, because of the Pritikin Program. And so I really feel that the Lord has used Nathan in a very mighty way, not only in my life but in the life of thousands and thousands of people. Millions of people, probably, around the world.

"I try to follow the program as best I can," he says, "probably ninety-eight or ninety-nine percent of the time. When I travel, my secretary, Kathy, notifies people that I am on the Pritikin Program." Again the odd word emphasis; this time it's on the word *am*. "She explains it's a very special diet and exercise program and they always go out of their way to provide the right type of foods. It gives me a chance not only to eat right and exercise right but also to introduce these other people to a new way of life. Kathy gives them very direct guidelines. In fact, if they want, she'll even send them some menus.

"I used to carry food with me when I traveled, but now the only thing I usually carry is oats. It's the easiest thing. At one time, I carried rice, but then you always have to prepare the rice. In fact when I go to Mt. Ararat, I usually have several bags of oats that I carry up on the mountain." He pauses a moment and explains, "I don't cook it, I just eat it raw. Some people like to cook it, but it gets a little slimy."

I asked Jim what he eats at home and whether, when he first went on the Pritikin Program, there was a separate menu for him and one for the rest of the family.

"Yes, there was originally," he remembers, "but now they're all getting around more to the Pritikin way. Mary would fix meat occasionally, and occasionally I would have chicken or fish, although I probably shouldn't because my cholesterol still stays pretty high.

"You see," he goes on, "I'm hyperlipidemic—Nathan had told me that—so even when I don't take any cholesterol in, I'm very lucky if I can get my blood levels down to 190, 180. My system just naturally produces cholesterol. So I *should* be totally vegetarian." (Hyperlipidemia is a genetic disposition to high lipid (fat) levels in the blood. Combined with excessive ingestion of fat and cholesterol, it can produce the high levels of blood cholesterol that in turn contribute to heart disease.)

"Typically," says Jim, "I have oats for breakfast with fruit, and for lunch, I'll probably have some soup and maybe some fruit. In the evening I just have vegetables, usually with rice. I have skim milk with my oats; that's the only dairy product I consume regularly. I might have lowfat cottage cheese occasionally. I guess I get that from time to time on airlines. I always ask for the vegetarian, low-cholesterol plate when I fly, although I think the safest thing for me to ask for is just a fruit plate."

"And to drink?" I asked.

"Just water," he replies. "Sometimes I'll have some juice."

Remembering Jim's description of his former diet and his enjoyment of rich foods, I asked what strategies he now uses to adhere to such a radically refined diet. Not a second is wasted in his reply. "My taste buds have changed," he says. "Now I can appreciate the simple foods, even vegetables; except that I'm still not at the point where I like carrots that much. In fact in my diet instructions I tell them to leave off the carrots.'' He laughs warmly, getting quite a kick out of his distaste for Bugs Bunny's favorite vegetable. ''Otherwise everybody feeds me carrots. I love rice and I love all the vegetables. And I love fruit. I guess my favorite meal would be just raw oats and fruit. I could eat that three times a day. I love it; I really love it.

''It's also a matter of discipline, though,'' he continues, leaning forward in his chair and then settling back again. ''I have to exercise discipline at every meal, every day. You have to take every day a step at a time. Every day is a new day, and if you've made a mistake the day before, you ignore it and say, 'This is a new day and I want to live it right. I want to follow the program.' '' He hesitates and snaps the thought shut, ''I realize that some days I do make mistakes and I might take something in that I shouldn't.''

I asked if that's how he manages to stay on the program as strictly as he does—by taking it one day at a time.

There is a long pause, as he seems to ponder the question very carefully. ''Yes,'' he answers, ''because if you look further ahead, like a week or two weeks . . .''

''It could become overwhelming?'' I suggested.

He nods, extends the proposition a bit further. ''You'd be asking yourself the question, 'I'm going to eat like this for the rest of my life?' But I realize it's a program I should be on as long as I'm here. God has told us that we are his temple, that he wants us to take care of this temple so he can live within us. He's given us that responsibility and if we take it really seriously, perhaps it makes it even easier for us to live a regimented life, a disciplined life.''

Our chairs have become hard and my tea cold. We decide to stretch for a break. Jim rounds up some brochures on his next trip to Turkey and the continuing search for Noah's Ark. Kathy delivers a few more messages. I inspect the citations on the wall—official seals and photographs from the moon flight. After another ten minutes, we're back in our chairs.

I asked Jim about any weaknesses that might tempt him to fall off the diet.

''Well, I might have a dessert,'' he answers tentatively.

''What kind?'' I pressed.

''I don't know,'' he answers with a pang, then drawls roundly, ''they're all so . . '' He laughs and I join him. This, the first genuinely light moment in what has up until now been a very deliberate and weighty conversation, opens the door a crack to the observation of Jim Irwin as a man of considerable wit and charm—and someone in possession of a keen sense of humor about himself. "They're all good," he laughs comfortably.

As Jim describes his goal of a regimented, disciplined life, I stifle the stereotypical image these words suggest—a life lacking in pleasure, nose to the grindstone, plodding along day after difficult day. It does not appear, however, that this is Jim Irwin's style. "No," he agrees. "I guess it's maybe . . . it's not even a balanced life; it's maybe a controlled life. I believe that each person should have control or charge over his or her life. I think we truly are the product of what we take in. That's certainly true in a physical sense and also in a spiritual sense, and even a mental sense. What we allow to come into our bodies will in every way influence the quality of life that we enjoy.

"So I guess from that standpoint," he continues further, "I like to exercise a certain amount of discipline in what I should eat, the amount of exercise I should do, where I spend my time, how I spend my time. We don't even have a television in our home because I think you can get carried away with that and spend too much very unproductive time with it, maybe even very destructive time. So I think we have to look at all the things on which we spend our time and decide if that's really what we should be doing."

Jim says he enjoys life *more* now that his experiences have given him the opportunity to ponder its meaning more. "I think," he says, "all of us come to a realization—sometimes it's late in life—that we're only here for a short period of time. When I was younger I thought life would be forever. Now I realize that life is just about over. My question to myself is 'What am I going to do, with the few remaining years, to really enjoy life to the utmost and get the most out of every waking hour, every sleeping hour?' Personally, I've come to the realization that probably the greatest pleasure, the greatest satisfaction, is in giving to other people—because I have taken so much. I've lived a very selfish life," he continues thoughtfully, "and now it's my turn to give back to others. One thing I can give them, share with them, is the Pritikin Program, which has really blessed me and with which they can really have an improved state of life."

I asked Jim if enjoyment of life and being productive are synonymous, considering that for many people enjoyment of life may involve things that in his mind are not necessarily desirable—lazy vacations, overeating, no exercise. I suggest that considering work enjoyable may be a perplexing proposition for many people.

Concurring, he amplifies the thought. "It's probably true that a lot of people don't enjoy what they're doing, don't enjoy their work and look at it simply as drudgery. It's something they have to do to make money, so that's probably why they eat: They come home and eat out of boredom . . ."

I wanted to know if he thought a lot of our excesses are a result of boredom or frustration.

"Yes," he acknowledges. "Because we don't feel satisfied with life as it's treating us; we believe somehow we might be able to get back at life by finding enjoyment in excess, indulging in food that we shouldn't have . . ." Again the idea trails off and he selects another, with more expansive implications: "But if somehow we could let people know that they will have ultimate satisfaction out of life by knowing that, if they follow the right program, they really do have control." A faint glow of passion begins to illuminate his speech. "I believe," he says, continuing his way over suppositions that seem to have sustained recurrent scrutiny, "the decisions we make will determine the quality of the life we live. And that affects all of life. The decision about what you are going to eat, how you're going to do exercise, what you are going to believe—they alter your life."

I wondered about his statement that he has led a selfish life. "Oh," he reflects softly, "I was taking a lot from life and not putting anything back." He offers to explain. "I was living to fly high and fast for most of life. I was leading a selfish existence, just for me, just for Jim Irwin so he could fly high-performance airplanes, fly spacecraft. But after I came back to the earth. I asked myself, 'What are you going to do after you've been to the moon?' What can I possibly do with my life that would provide satisfaction, challenge? I think we all have to do that sometime."

Remembering his description of his intense absorption in the space program, I asked if he has gone back and renewed relationships with people he might have slighted during those years.

"Oh, I'm still working on my relationships with people," he answers candidly. "Particularly my wife." Having worked hard to develop her own conclusions about the meaning of life, Mary Irwin has joined Jim in his work at High Flight and sometimes travels with him. He expresses appreciation and satisfaction at Mary's support of his new-found mission.

I asked about the children.

"I was away a lot of the time while they were growing up," he admits, "but we've come into a closer relationship. Two of the girls are married now. In fact, we're grandparents now. They've kind of stepped out into their own lives, but we're close. We all try to do things together as a family." He pauses and corrals a memory. "It was neat when we had the dedication of our grandson recently. All the kids came in for it. A daughter and her husband came in from New York and another daughter and her boyfriend came from California. That was a neat experience.''

Considering Jim's concern about the potential effects of his illness on the kind of continued active life he envisions for himself, I asked if when he was recuperating from his heart attacks or even the bypass surgery, he had seriously evaluated what his life might be like, if he had reviewed his life's direction intellectually, perhaps emotionally.

''Well,'' he says casually, tampering with the intent of my question, ''at that point I really didn't know how long I'd be around. I certainly didn't think I'd be able to do anything very active. That bothered me, because I've always been very active. And I wondered if I'd ever be able to fly again. Even now I still haven't been able to get a medical certificate back. But I'm trying. The only flying I do now is sometimes with a hang glider or an ultralight, which you can do without having a medical certificate.''

''Do you miss it?'' I asked.

''No-o-o,'' he answers, ''not that much, because I'm so busy doing other things. I guess it was—and still is—a matter of prestige or ego that I could fly on my own if it were necessary.''

''When you read Pritikin's book, were you desperate or did you read it more out of curiosity?''

''Well, I knew that what I had been doing with the nutritionist was probably not the right approach,'' he says flatly. ''And of course after the second attack, I did discover the importance of a lowered level of cholesterol, and Nathan's book went along with that in a very dramatic way. So I said to myself, 'Why just reduce cholesterol, like the conventional wisdom suggests? If you want to get maximum benefit and improvement in a short period of time, why not just cut it out completely?'

''I was looking for the answer,'' he concedes in a definitive tone. ''I was more open to considering all possibilities by that time. I thought the Lord had given me several nudges, some good warnings that I'd better heed, otherwise I wouldn't be around very long. So I decided that Nathan's book really did make sense. Since then, I have had the opportunity to go through the full program. They invited me to come back and meet with each group of participants at the Colorado Health Center, to tell my story and encourage people. And I have done that with all the Pritikin centers.''

He stirs, starts to rearrange his pad and pen, finally lays the pad on the chair he's been using for an armrest. ''I guess I'm a little distressed on every visit,'' he begins. ''You see people who are in such b-a-a-d shape through neglect, at least that's what I can judge on outward appearance. They're obese, so many of them, and they've never been active physically, or at least since they were very young children. I can understand that they're searching to turn back the clock, to give themselves some hope for quality of life. It's a little distressing when you look at the population at the Pritikin centers because it's like looking at a microcosm of the population of the United States.

"These people are victims of the good life," he continues, "and look what the good life has done for us. I'll be the first one to speak out on that because I'm a victim of the so-called good life. We have so much to make it easy for us, so many temptations that it's hard to live a regimented, disciplined life, a simple life-style. It's a tragedy that we who are supposed to have a so-called advanced civilization are so uncivilized, really."

His words on this subject come unhurriedly and easily. "I think it's a result of lack of information," he says. "Lack of motivation. Lack of will. Lack of discipline. I enjoy going to all those centers and encouraging people because I get positive feedback. They kind of encourage me as I encourage them. I think you need a lot of mutual support to follow a program such as Pritikin. But I always suggest to my friends that they just take a month out of their life and challenge themselves to follow the program very strictly. Because I think that at the end of twenty-six days or even maybe even thirteen days, they will feel so much better. They will be convinced that they will have a better life, maybe an extended life, but certainly a better quality."

He leans back in his chair, stretching from side to side, the pen still in his hand. "I've always said I don't long to have an extended life but as long as I'm here I want to be able to make a positive contribution, and I think that the Pritikin Program will allow me to do that. I feel better; I think better."

I suggest that such a dramatic change can be scary for some people.

"Yes," he says, "many people, I guess, like to be dependent on a doctor's care and, maybe, medication. I think that we've all become very drug dependent. I was on so many medications as a result of my heart attacks . . . ." He quickly expands the focus of his thought. "Unfortunately most of us will not change our habits until our life is threatened. Unfortunately, when you wait that long you might not be able to regain the quality of life."

"Do you think," I wondered, "there might be a connection between a person's psychological state of mind and a disease affecting him? You were speaking before about how hectic your life was, because you had so many obligations. Were you implying a stress factor in what happened to you health-wise?''

"I believe that the way we think will affect the way our body functions. I don't think you can separate those. The actions within our brain will control other actions within the body. We know that. But it's whether we think about them in a positive or a negative way that's important. There is a feedback, and I'm convinced that life is more than just the body. Life is more than just what you can see and touch. But sometimes it's difficult to get the right balance between all of these.

"You know," he summarizes, "I had the health problems since I came back to the earth. I had financial problems. I thought the Lord was finished with me, teaching me lessons, then . . .''

"You have a hard head, Jim," I interject. We both laugh. Again some of the Irwin Irish charm begins to cavort among our serious words. "I'm glad I have a hard head," he grins. "Look what happened to me on Mt. Ararat." He is comfortable telling the story. "I was knocked unconscious. I spent the night all alone on the mountain, unconscious for six hours. I told everyone else in my group never to travel alone on the mountain and here I disregarded those instructions. I was looking for a short cut, a quick descent, and I must have been hit on the head by a rock that knocked me out. Fortunately I still had my backpack with my sleeping bag in it. It was a miracle that I became conscious just as it was getting dark, and that I still had my sleeping bag available. I was able to get into the sleeping bag and have some warmth that night. Otherwise I would have frozen to death. I didn't have any pain and I didn't have any concerns because I figured they'd find me the next morning. Except," he adds facetiously, "I didn't know what condition I'd be in when they found me.

"A doctor friend told me later that I was lucky I didn't sever my arteries. It's easy to bleed from scalp wounds and I had some deep scalp wounds. In fact they had to shave off all of my hair to stitch up my scalp. They did it at a Turkish hospital. It was thirty hours from the time I had the accident until they did the surgery. They said, 'Boy, you're lucky you're in good shape.' I told them it was because I was on the Pritikin Program. So," Jim chuckles briefly, still serious, "the Pritikin Program not only gets you high but allows you to go through some serious accidents and still come back. Three weeks after that accident, three weeks to the day, I was back on the mountain continuing the search, even though I'd lost a lot of blood and wasn't at peak strength.

"It's my hard Irish head," he concludes and then adds smartly as we both laugh, "and my Irish luck."

I ask Irishman Irwin if he ever does any drinking.

"Oh, occasionally," he answers. "But I have to be careful now that I'm on the Pritikin Program. I don't think I ever used alcohol to excess, and I drink occasionally now, but usually just white wine. Rarely would I have a beer. I don't think alcohol is good for you, so I try to stay away from it." He pauses as he considers what he's just said. "I find that when I drink, even a glass of wine, it relaxes me so much that I lose my discipline and then I'm inclined to eat things that I shouldn't be eating. What it amounts to," he summarizes, "is that it starts from those decisions you make. So if you can resist that first impulse . . ."

"How do you do that?" I ask.

"I have to prepare myself ahead of time." Either I look skeptical or he realizes that his tone is overly serious and dour. He grins, widely this time, his smile warming the room. "I just reinforce myself. I say, 'Here you're going into this situation and there might be a temptation there, but, Jim, this is your opportunity to be strong . . . and resist it.' " Again he laughs at himself and the occasional futility of it all.

"Does it work?" I prodded.

"Most times it does. Sometimes I do weaken though. My biggest weakness would probably be dessert. I know it's not good for you, but I guess the rationalization is 'I've worked so hard today—I've run for an hour, maybe I've run six or seven miles. My system can accommodate it.' " Abruptly Irwin's voice changes from amiable and easy-going, as he enjoys a moment of amusement about himself, to the very considered tone in which he delivers the coda to this thought. "But that's foolish," he says, and is suddenly quiet.

When I asked further about the need for support from people close to him, he answers immediately, "I think you need support; there's no doubt about that. And it helps very much if your spouse supports the program. I don't think it's necessary that he or she eats the same way, just so they support it and encourage you. I know if I deviated very far from it, my wife would remind me, 'Oh, you're going off the Pritikin Program?' "

I asked Jim what advice he'd give to people attempting a life-style change such as the one he's made.

He thinks a moment. "I guess," he says, "that every day is a day of fresh commitment, just like a renewal of your spirit. You wake up in the morning and the first thing you say to yourself is 'I'm on the Pritikin Program today; yesterday I was on it'—hopefully you were on it yesterday." Again demonstrating his awareness of the difficulties of maintaining a strict life-style change, he issues another one of those shallow belly laughs he seems to prefer, coming up short, more airy than robust. " 'Maybe,' " he continues with his self-advice, " 'I didn't do so well yesterday, but today I'm on it again and I'm going to do better today than I did yesterday. I'm going to follow that program.' I think," he concludes, "it becomes easier each day."

For Irwin, getting the exercise he requires has become an integral part of his life, even while keeping his heavy traveling schedule. "I've come to the point where I enjoy exercise," he says. "I look forward to it and if for some reason I miss it, I feel like I've been cheated. So the next day," he laughs, "I might go out and do it twice as long.

"I usually run or jog; I go six, seven miles. But if the weather's really miserable, I just get on my stationary bike and ride for an hour to try to get my heart rate to the same point as when I jog. I enjoy the jogging time, because, for me, it's a time when I can really relax. When I'm at home and on the bike, I have the telephone right next to me and I'm reading. But when I'm out jogging, I have time to meditate, to pray, to be completely myself, to get my life better organized. Usually when I travel, my secretary will tell my hosts that I like to run, and many people like to run with me."

Remembering the rigidity he describes as important to his fitness routines, I ask him if he runs at certain times every day.

"No," he answers, "I'm flexible. Sometimes when it's nice, I go out from the office. I change my clothes and run up the canyon. There are some beautiful areas up there. At home I run around the neighborhood. When I'm on the road, I try to run in the morning. If I get my running done in the morning, the whole day is downhill. I feel like I have it behind me and I feel so relaxed and good about myself."

"What's left that you haven't had a chance to do?"

"I would like to find Noah's Ark," he answers immediately. "I love to climb mountains, so I can be as happy on Mt. Ararat—where we've been looking—as I am in the Rockies."

It would appear that the heavens—whether on foot or by airplane—release a feeling of freedom in Jim Irwin, as well as provide opportunities to nurture his constant search for his personal limits. I wonder if he would attempt to climb a mountain like Everest.

"I don't know," he responds and then thinks about it. "You know, when Dick Bass climbed Everest and was the oldest man to do it at fifty-five, I thought, 'Well, man, I can't beat that record now.' I guess I could do it next year at fifty-six," he laughs. "The only reason I climb Mt. Ararat is that I hope that might produce evidence of the ark. Then I'd like to find the Ark of the Covenant. We're also involved in trying to find the exact exodus route the children of Israel followed from Egypt.

"But," he muses, "I've taken care of most of my projects. I thought when I came back from the moon that I should take the message I understood in space to two places especially—Northern Ireland and the Soviet Union. And I've done that. I've only been to the Soviet Union once, but I've been back almost every year to Ireland since I recovered from the first heart attack—because my father was Irish and I was born on St. Patrick's Day. That's why I took a shamrock to the moon and left it there."

I ask Jim if, when he was on the moon, he was enlightened about the source of his childhood dream of exploring space.

"No," he answers, "I still don't know why I should happen to have that feeling as a little kid growing up in Pittsburgh. Maybe the Lord just put that desire in me—to go into the sky, to go into space, to go to the moon. But I got to it through a weird set of circumstances, many of which were contrary to my purpose—setbacks." He thinks a moment. "That's why it still amazes me that it worked out the way it did . . . I think there was a lot of divine intervention. I sense now that God prepared me through a set of what people would call tragedies."

"You've talked about what space has given to you. What about the rest of us?"

"Well, I think there's hope that space exploration will give something to everyone. One of the fallouts from space technology, for example, has been excellent communications, so we can know instantly what happens worldwide. And the space shuttle is a more economical form of transportation. The next step is the space station, where people can live and work for a long period of time. We'll have factories in space." As he speaks, he breathes a small chuckle that suggests not all of Jim Irwin's space-exploring days are over. "It would be easier on your heart in space. It would just be the stress of getting there and back. In fact," he confirms, "I volunteered to go on another flight as a former heart patient and also a chaplain and former astronaut—on a space station or maybe a moon or Mars base. We've just taken the first step in space, but we've already seen a tremendous potential.

"We will not only continue to explore space," he goes on, "but we'll begin to use it, as we're using the space around the earth—to form products that you could never form on earth, to be able to look at the earth and understand it better, from a different perspective, a total perspective. To somehow preserve the earth, preserve our quality of life."

A spark gleams in Jim's eyes as he speaks about his space experiences and their significance for his life; his evenly modulated voice takes on an edge, an excitement. "I think space has given us the opportunity to see ourselves from far away and to realize that the earth is special. It's the only natural home for man that we know of in the entire universe and we'd better take care of it. And we'd better take care of one another, if we're to continue our journey through space.

"As astronauts, moving away from earth, we can see it and realize how precious it is. Logically, we're then obligated to take care of it; we are stewards of the earth. In the Pritikin Program, we . . . look at our own life . . . and realize, 'You know, life is short but here's something I can do . . . that will extend my life, will add quality to it.' And so participating in the Pritikin Program gives us a new perspective on our individual life.

"I think that one of our problems," he suggests, "is that we don't love ourselves enough, and if we can't love ourselves, we can't love others, so we can't be concerned about them. At High Flight, we want people to be not only prepared for life, but also prepared for death. Because the time will come when all of us have to leave. What's going to happen then? Where are we going to go?"

Jim's question implies that he considers some places more desirable than others. He pauses a moment, sneaks out a wide grin and then says with another shallow Irwin laugh, "I guess I think about that more than I did before." Then he adds, "I'm convinced that there is life after death and and I want to go to the very best place."

The light mood quickly changes and Jim says somberly, "I think the part that gives me the greatest satisfaction is being able to make an impact on other people's lives and see that their lives are changed, that we share something in common. That they have new appreciation for the earth, an appreciation for life—a new zest."

Today

Today Jim Irwin lives in Colorado with Mary, his wife of twenty-six years, and his family. The pace he continues to keep would challenge even a much younger man free of any debilitating disease. The High Flight Foundation provides the integral link between the insights of Jim's past experiences and his present commitments. "It's a Christian foundation," says Jim, "whose purpose is to lift people to a better way of life through a spiritual dimension. We named it High Flight after a poem by that name written by an RAF pilot who died in World War I. And I had a high flight going into space, and we want everyone to have a high flight as they live their lives, to have the very best life they could possibly have.

"I have three other retired astronauts who work with me in the foundation. We go out and we speak in schools, trying to encourage young people in their pursuit of excellence, trying to motivate them, trying to inspire them, trying to help them find some direction to their lives. Many of them are interested in space, and maybe when they hear firsthand about our experiences, they'll be more motivated and see a new direction, a new purpose to their lives. We call it Project Uplift."

By his own estimation, Jim travels twenty days out of each month to share the message of his Apollo flight. Many of his trips are packed with one- or two-day stops at which he lectures to various groups. Others involve sustained visits, such as his frequent trips to China. In addition, in recent years, he has mounted an annual expedition to the Middle East to search for the religious artifacts he feels have significance for contemporary life. Expedition members carry their own supplies and equipment, and camp at the base of the mountain. The expedition is so strenuous that the brochure advertising it carries the following disclaimer: "Participation will be limited to persons free of any physical handicap, and we reserve the right to exclude anyone not in good health or not physically fit." Quite a load for a patient with heart disease.

Aside from these activities, Irwin also accepts occasional invitations to visit the various Pritikin centers and share his experiences with participants. In fact, I first met him when he made a day trip from Colorado Springs to Los Angeles to speak at a symposium of the Pritikin Research Foundation.

Astronaut Irwin is now completely free of the medication prescribed to combat the effects of his heart disease, even the aspirin recommended as a blood thinner. When asked about being under a doctor's care for continued monitoring of his health, he answered nonchalantly, "Well, I guess the only thing would be NASA," referring to his annual Houston physical and health evaluation—an unusually cavalier attitude for a man who has suffered multiple heart attacks and bypass surgery.

Aside from his daily five- to six-mile run, or, in bad weather, an hourly ride on his stationary bicycle, Irwin continues to test his physical limits by hiking in the local Colorado mountains, climbing Pikes Peak, for example. "The first summer I went on the Pritikin Program," he remembers, "I was able to climb Pikes Peak again. When I got to the top of the mountain, I was jogging—at 14,000 feet. That was something I could never do, even as a young adult. When I'd get to high altitude—even though I loved to climb mountains—when I'd get up there, I was laboring. I just felt exhausted. But now, to have that type of resource—that I can get to the top of Pikes Peak and jog—I'm considering doing the race to Pikes Peak.''

Added to his Rocky Mountain outings, Jim has routinely made the difficult ascent to the top of 17,000-foot Mt. Ararat in Turkey (the site of his fall and his subsequent head injury) to continue his search for Noah's Ark. ''We're looking primarily on Mt. Ararat,'' he explains, ''because there've been sightings of what looks like an ark up there near the ice cap. So we've been looking around the edge of the ice cap. It's a big ice cap, almost twenty-three square miles. And it's at high altitude and the weather is very changeable. We've tried to do it in a very systematic way—taking different areas of the mountain to look at—and this year we will have some more sophisticated, high technology equipment that can penetrate rocks and ice to see if we might be able to locate any remains.''

Because of his bypass surgery, Irwin has not yet received his recertification as a pilot but he continues to hope that the FAA will change its position. In the meantime, there is much work to be done spreading the word of his ''High Flight.''

''It was interesting,'' says Jim, ''just after we found the white rock on the moon. I looked over my shoulder and there was a beautiful green rock. We brought that back with us also, and they say it's probably more important than the white rock. It appears to be about half a billion years older than the white rock, the so-called Genesis rock. So it's really the oldest material returned from the moon.'' He pauses and then repeats, ''The green rock''— an appropriate discovery for a hardheaded Irish astronaut who has dared life at seemingly every juncture and who has the knack—and the faith—to turn adversity into opportunity, despair into incentive and defeat into a mission for the future.

And so, for astronaut Col. James Irwin, the challenges continue.

Chapter 3

Jack Rutta, 60, stockbroker. Married, two grown children.

Heart attack, triple bypass surgery.

Diagnosis: coronary artery disease.

I

"Your body's such a wonderful machine, why resent something that can help it?"

In the early '60s, a physician working in the field of cardiac care perfected a surgical technique that was destined to be widely used, save many lives and generate a sustained flurry of controversy from both within and without the medical profession. The procedure is deceptively simple. A section of superfluous vein is removed from a patient's leg by one member of a team of surgeons. Another surgeon grafts this vein onto one of the major coronary arteries of the patient's heart to "bypass" the blockage that led to the heart attack and to insure a clean flow of blood and nutrients to his heart muscle. (New procedures also utilize the internal mammary artery that runs along the wall of the chest.)

Coronary bypass surgery—as this procedure is known—was performed on an estimated 200,000 Americans in 1984, at a total cost of some five billion dollars. The procedure, developed by Dr. Rene G. Favaloro at the Cleveland Clinic and sometimes referred to colloquially as open-heart surgery, is actually performed on the arteries that lie on the surface of the heart. Perhaps the misnomer results from the fact that the operation requires a large incision, laying open the chest cavity, and snipping the patient's ribs. Throughout the surgery, the patient is maintained on a heart-lung machine, allowing the surgical team free access to the heart. The response of the patient's heart to removal from the heart-lung machine—requiring the heart to function on its own again—is generally considered an indication of the individual's postoperative prognosis. In some cases, it can take hours to wean the patient off the machine, to get his heart pumping and have him breathing on his own again.

Controversy continues concerning the medical establishment's enthusiastic support of this innovative surgical procedure. Some critics consider that far too many bypass procedures are performed based on the limited criteria that the patient has experienced a heart attack or the chest pain referred to as angina. Others worry that bypass surgery is often too successful, inducing a false sense of security among heart patients and a tendency to disregard suggestions for a modified lifestyle. It remains, however, that a great number of people have been aided by bypass surgery, and many are perhaps alive today because of it. Before the procedure was available, it's estimated that one of every six men who experienced angina—the chest pain associated with heart disease—was dead four years after the onset of symptoms. Of patients surviving heart attacks, nearly one in every five was dead at the end of four years. It seems doubtful that Alan Keiser would have survived had he not undergone a quadruple bypass. Although Jim Irwin implies some ambivalence regarding the necessity of his bypass surgery, as he explains, "At the time, I knew of no alternative."

Heart patients, in viewing the procedure as an easy way out of a difficult situation, have themselves made an inadvertent contribution to the development of bypass surgery's tarnished reputation. As we've seen, bypass surgery is not always a sure way out. Such was Nathan Pritikin's opinion, and so he sought to present his diet and exercise program as a more effective alternative. However, his radical position was not fully supported by his medical staff. Some tended to the opinion that there are indeed patients for whom bypass surgery is appropriate, but then *only* when combined with a postoperative life-style change.

A coronary bypass is not something to be taken lightly—either at the presurgical decision-making stage, or as Jim Irwin's experiences suggest, in the postoperative recuperation period. The following experiences of Jack Rutta, combined with those of Fred Rizk presented in the next chapter, present two different sides to the bypass story. One man's wisdom induced him to accept bypass as a welcome inevitability and then to adhere strictly to a modified life-style. Another patient opted to seek other alternatives.

Jack Rutta and Fred Rizk are similar in many aspects. Both, by their own admission, are cast from a macho mold. Both are physically active—Rutta in sports, Rizk in big-game hunting. Both are proud of their virility and tend to express it in physical terms. Both are self-made men, fiercely independent, stubborn, persistent, capable of intense commitments. And both are afflicted with the need to influence the lives of others while being peculiarly unreceptive to help and guidance for themselves. Each man describes his personality as Type A—driven, relentless and hard on themselves, and both men engage in a chronic and not necessarily successful battle with the evasive spectre of their own self-awareness.

Two men, each faced with the prospect of coronary bypass surgery, each opting for a divergent solution. The story of how each man came to his respective decision and has coped with its effects is a study in two very disparate kinds of courage.

If you take the Santa Monica Freeway east from Beverly Hills and then, by the San Bernardino Freeway, head further east, you will eventually see a sign that directs you to Boyle Heights, or what is called East Los Angeles. Past downtown, which has sprawled south from its original location, past the freight yards and the warehouses, the freeway skirts the area, but comes close enough to allow a view of old three-story tenement buildings and small, compact single-family dwellings. Shingled and painted white, dirty now, they are laid out close together and snake their way up and down the shallow hills.

This is what is loosely called East L.A. The Boyle Heights area, which it encompasses, is close to the center of the original city of Los Angeles and like many inner cities, the area has bulged with wave after wave of immigrants. Today it strives to accommodate colonies from the south—Mexicans, El Salvadorans, stragglers from Guatemala. Years back it hosted Japanese and Russians, who emigrated to California looking for work, and Jews and American blacks who, lured by the promise of a new life in the soft glow of the California sun, came west from the eastern and southern United States.

Jack Rutta grew up on the outskirts of Boyle Heights. He remembers East L.A. fondly. "It was like a small town in the middle of a big city. I wasn't hemmed in at all. It was twenty-five percent Jewish, twenty-five percent Japanese, twenty-five percent Russian and twenty-five percent black. One of my most traumatic moments was in '42 when they took all the Japanese to the camps. We were the only family left in the apartment house. Here I was all alone; in an apartment house full of people, we were the only ones left. That was one of the first dramatic feelings I had. I kept wondering, 'Hey, what happened to them?' It was one of the first times I had the feeling of . . . of something gone awry. They were kicked out, all the people I grew up with.''

Jack's father had worked as a baker in the east until his lungs became clogged with flour, and he moved his family to Los Angeles with the hope of renewed health. Once settled, he started a junk collection business, depending on his son for help. Jack remembers, ''I brought home more than he did in a week. And I think that bothered him. I could carry a hundred pounds when I was a little punk under five-foot. I used to make six dollars a day. He made four. We had a route. We used to go to apartment buildings; we'd cultivate the Filipinos. I used to go by myself on Saturdays and Sundays when I was in high school.''

Jack left Boyle Heights after he returned from the service. ''The war,'' he says, ''moved things west.''

West was a whole different story. A sprawling land of suburbs— bungalows set back from tree-lined streets, lush green lawns, roofs and fences covered with flowering bougainvillea, a neat grid of boulevards and avenues, the thriving territory of postwar L.A. The prestigious addresses moved continually toward the ocean, from the area around MacArthur Park to the brick mansions and Spanish-style apartment buildings of Hancock Park, then the bungalows and ranch houses and small castles perched atop the hills above Hollywood. Finally it seemed to come to a temporary rest on the flatlands of Beverly Hills.

Jack Rutta moved with it. From an urban tangle of apartments, industrial buildings and commerce, from the congestion of the urban center to the freshness of the ocean breeze. From a multi-family tene- ment building to ''Paul Trousdale's house,'' the former residence of the man who developed most of the expensive homes in this very expensive part of town. Geographically, it was a move of a little over ten miles. But miles don't tell the story.

I originally met Jack Rutta at a farewell party for a middle- management executive at the corporate offices of California Federal Savings. Jack had stopped in on his way to his Thursday night square- dancing session. That intrigued me and we began to talk. Outwardly, Rutta looks like a typical corporate executive, even allowing for the half glasses that sit atop his nose occasionally. He's a compact man, about five feet, ten inches tall, has a strong build and carries himself with the air of someone who is used to sports or physical activity. My questions about how he got into square dancing led us to his easy revelation that he had gone on the Pritikin Program because of heart disease. We decided to talk.

Jack's office is on the ground floor of the California Federal Savings Building on the Miracle Mile section of Wilshire Boulevard. If miracles ever happened here, they have long ceased to exist and the area is now in need of a face-lift. Actually Jack has no office. He exercises squatter's rights on a corner of the bank lobby, a kind of free-form space that he has jammed full of necessary clutter—rate books, computer tapes, yellow pads, sales brochures. It's the type of arrangement that is often symptomatic of a thoroughly competent but cavalier approach to organization.

Once retired, Jack is now testing the waters again as a stockbroker for the savings association's investor program. He sits on a small secretarial chair and talks about the heart attack he had six years ago. He uses the chair unceremoniously, poised like a man who is sitting on the tailgate of a vehicle parked in the desert, watching for rabbits. I sit across from him, claiming a small space in the organized clutter for my notes and tape recorder.

I asked him first to describe his heart attack.

He leans back in the small armless chair and thinks for a moment about how to describe it. Although an easy man with words, Jack is not one to embellish a story for effect. He would be the last person you'd accuse of pumping air into his conversation, the last to attempt to con you into believing something he knows isn't true or is contrary to your own beliefs. He himself is skeptical by nature and demands proof.

"I was on the freeway," he begins, "and I started getting an uncomfortableness all the way down my left side, a tingling. There was no constriction. The bottom of my jaw was sore and my shoulders were sore.

"I pulled off the freeway at the La Cienega exit and drove into Kaiser Permanente [clinic]. I got out of my car and walked in and sat down. The guy behind the counter looked me over and then he asked me what was wrong. I told him, 'I don't think I feel well.' And so he didn't think I had just walked in off the street, I said, 'My wife has a card here.' He took a look at me and said, 'You've got something going on.' I agreed with him. I said, 'Yes, doctor.' Then they laid me down, and I told them, 'I have Blue Cross.' I had all my cards.

"The doctor, or whoever he was, said to me, 'You can stay here.' I told him, 'Well, OK, I'll stay here.' " Jack recounts the conversation easily. "It made sense," he explains. "Then I asked him, 'Would you be kind enough to call my wife, Edie?' "

I asked Jack if he was scared by all of this. There is a long pause after which he shakes his head no. Then he crosses his arms in front of his chest, goes back over it again and says, "I don't know. Everybody asks me that question, but I can't answer it." He thinks it over again and says finally, "I was not scared."

Jack claims he is unaware of any emotional reaction during that time. "I was very analytical," he says. "I was looking around. I was very into what was going on. By then, I knew what it was. They were moving too fast. I saw them taking my blood pressure and I saw the other things they were doing, and I said to myself, 'OK, I understand.' " He pauses for a moment, anticipating my next question. "I suspected something was not right in the car. But I'm too dumb to be scared. Nothing . . . no physical person scares me. I've done things that afterward I sit back and wonder why I did them."

As if expecting a further question, he answers it with one of his own. "Do I know what fear is? Yes, I have to say that," he concedes, delivering the short admission in a tone that indicates he's not interested in discussing the subject further. But I decide to pursue it, suspecting that whatever fear Jack Rutta might have felt under the circumstances was suppressed, an option he acknowledges he has been known to exercise regarding his other emotions. I asked if he could describe what fear looks like to him, if perhaps he could think of an example of a fearful situation.

The question throws him slightly. With no pat answer, he mulls it over. "A fearful situation?" he asks himself, and then says, as if he's willing to accommodate the request, "Let me think of a fearful situation." His eyes search the plate-glass windows in front of him for an image. I'm suddenly conscious of the noise level in the room—the voices of customers and tellers, phones constantly ringing and the clatter of computer printers.

Finally Jack latches on to something. "It was in New Caledonia, while in the service," he starts. "I was attached to Naval Intelligence. The Vichy French were out there and somebody reported they were broadcasting to the Japanese. I spotted the location and we went in to investigate. We knew they were transmitting—you could see the transmitter—and it was obvious that someone had to go in there and close it up. I was thinking through what we were going to do, listening to all these geniuses around me, and I thought to myself, 'Who in the hell wants to go down there and do that kind of crap? I'm not going to do it.' I think I was scared then," he says thoughtfully.

"Of what?" I asked. "The fact you might die?"

"I don't know; I just think I was scared," he muses and picks at another thought. "I don't dream," he says, "at least I don't think I do, but I know of one dream I have. Golden tweezers are coming at my eyes, plucking something out. Tweezers, gold tweezers. G-o-o-o-ld, absolutely gold," he emphasizes. "Plucking something out. In Pennsylvania when I was a year old, my dad's car went off the road and I got cut. They had to put some stitches in the cut, and then they pulled them out with gold tweezers. That's the only dream I'm aware of. It's a funny dream. A scared kid? I don't know. That's the only other memory I have of fear.''

His next thought brings us directly back to the present. ''My wife, Edie, got mad at me the other day. I saw a guy picking on a car that was parked by the music center, where we were going. It was seven o'clock on a Sunday. I told Edie, 'Go on in.' And I just walked over to him and said, 'Hey buster . . . take off.' Afterwards she said to me, 'You can't do that.' And I said to her, 'Edie, I've done it many times.' '' He sits back and waits for the effect.

He then goes on to describe another incident: ''I'm driving down Grandview Boulevard. I see a private car with a red light on it. I couldn't understand it, so I stopped my car. There was a young lady in another car and two guys get out of the car with the red light on it. I got out of my own car and confronted them. One guy warned me not to interfere. He looked at me and said, 'Who are you?' I asked him, 'Who are you that you've got a red light on?' I didn't think he was a cop. He said to me, 'I'm a police officer.' I responded, 'Fine, let's see your badge.' He said, 'I don't have a badge,' and I said to him, 'Let's see your goddamn badge before I go at you.' That's me,'' Jack concludes. ''You shouldn't do things like that, but I do. I don't know why.''

Inspired now, he completes his train of thought, ''Maybe I should have been the guy on the white charger—justice shall prevail, morals and all that stuff.''

I ask him what happened on the day of the heart attack after they admitted him to the hospital. ''Oh,'' he answers sprightly. ''After they got me stabilized—setup—I called my doctor. He told me, 'As long as you're resting and you're OK, stay there. But let's get you an angiogram. You just lie there and I'll call Jerry.' Jerry,'' explains Jack, ''was the heart specialist.''

Kaiser Permanente, where Jack remained after his heart attack, is a full-service membership health-care clinic and hospital. Members pay an annual fee and are provided with whatever health services they require. The hospital admitted Jack to its coronary-care unit because his wife was a member. He stayed in the hospital for two weeks after the attack. During that time his doctor requested an angiogram to determine the extent of his heart damage and the degree of artery blockage. Because he had had some damage to his heart tissue as a result of the attack, his doctor and the consulting cardiologist decided to allow Jack time to recover from the attack before considering bypass surgery. With all these things in mind, I asked him what he thought about when he was in the hospital.

Jack looks at me as if I've just asked for a dissertation on the state of the American economy, a discussion he'd probably be better prepared to present. "Nothing," he says. "My children came by to see me. Edie was by, my friends came by. I told them all, 'Hey, nothing ever happens to Jack.' I never had another thought." Then without any prodding, he says strongly, "I'll follow that philosophy until the day somebody hits me over the head with a club. Nothing's ever going to happen to me."

"I didn't feel bad," he continues. "I wasn't running around, but I had all my motion and everything. It was just that there was damage done wherever that thing occurred . . . the doctor tried to explain it to me. He said, 'There's different coloration in there and we're going to have to do bypass but you have to heal up a little.' "

Unlike most people, Jack Rutta had had a kind of "warning" about a potential heart problem, what he describes as a hot feeling in his chest. "Years before, I had started getting, as I call it, the hot esophagus. I won't call it constriction. It usually happened after excess exercise. I used to play ball at the time, baseball and softball. I was always in good shape—never was heavy or anything. But after running too much, there would be a hot sensation in the esophagus, and I knew something was different. It started, I guess, when I was forty years old or thereabouts. It was nothing severe. I would just stop for a minute and it would go away."

Although it would be tempting to describe Jack's hot pain as a precursor to full-fledged angina, and thus an indication of heart disease, it is more likely that the sensation he describes was the result of an irritated trachea, probably from the two-plus-packs-a-day cigarette habit he had developed. Such an irritation would become more pronounced when there was an increased demand for air, during exercise for example, and might well produce a hot sensation in the esophagus, which lies directly under the trachea. The same feeling might also have been the result of heartburn—acid from the stomach reflected up the esophagus. The fact that Jack's hot esophagus might not have been a direct symptom of heart disease is irrelevant to his story, however, because the discomfort alerted him to the possibility that something was wrong and caused him to take steps to avert it.

"Although I had always been very active, I was working as a stockbroker then, sitting in the office doing nothing. My diet was right—or so I thought. I was always in so-called good shape. I didn't need to work out to be in good shape in those days," he adds as an aside. "But that's when it started and all I did was tell my doctor about it. He told me, 'It's very simple, Jack. You don't have to pitch a whole game against the kids.' " He stops to explain, "You see, every July Fourth I used to pitch a ball game against the all-stars of the Pony League. Everybody looked forward to it. I could always go the four innings, that didn't bother me. I never had any discomfort in those games. Maybe it was because I enjoyed them. I don't know. So all I did back then," he recalls, "was to just forget about it."

Jack was in his early forties when he started experiencing what he calls his hot esophagus, which was, for him, a potential warning of his heart condition. By then he had married his childhood sweetheart and had initiated the succession of businesses that would eventually make him financially successful. He and his first wife, Judy, established a life-style not dissimilar to Alan and Bea Keiser's—Jack worked hard to make his family comfortable, while Judy "raised the kids."

Jack describes his life easily, communicating a feeling of accomplishment and satisfaction. "We were in a fairly nice middle-income group," he says. "We had friends. When I say friends, we had four, you know, friends—the same group that grew up together on the east side of town, the kind of friends you can count on. There was no divorce in that group. We were all lucky—the affluence was fairly nice."

He gets up, takes off his suit coat and puts it over the back of his desk chair, then comes back and sits on his perch. "Today I think I could call on any of them or anyone could call on me. It was a good background, a good way to grow up. I was very fortunate with my kids—never had any doubt about them. My wife really raised them. I was 'what made Sammy run,' you know. Besides being a stockbroker, I owned a money-order company, I owned car washes. Judy and I always traveled once a year; we always took a vacation. And as the kids got older, she went back to teaching."

"Are you a workaholic?" I asked.

"Yes," he answers tersely. "I have always been a workaholic. I would work maybe twenty hours a day and the only time I ever missed a day of work was when I had a hernia operation."

"And were you the leader of your group?"

"Yes," he answers easily, "I guess so. Judy and I were a hub. Their youngsters all grew up in our house. Our friends," he discloses, "respected my judgment.'

Jack recites the litany of his life as if he is well pleased. He is, in many ways, a comfortable individual. He seems at ease with himself. The lines on his face suggest he has spent more time smiling in optimism than frowning in despair. His eyes are sharp and lively and he looks directly at you when he speaks. His hair is graying but still retains a hint of what looks like auburn color. He's a careful dresser—the shirt a subtle match with the suit and always the complementary tie—his suits usually in shades of brown and tan. But for all the fastidiousness, he also conveys an impression of spontaneity and casual masculine assurance. He invites conversation and seems to inspire confidence among friends and clients alike.

Asked if he ever thought about the role stress or pressure play in heart disease, he answers without a moment's hesitation. "Yes, but at the time I started having the hot esophagus I had a pretty successful brokerage firm. So there was no lack of money. I had no debt to speak of in those days. There were no financial stresses of any kind. I was never compulsive about my goals. They just came—the financial rewards."

He pauses for a moment, looks around the room as if to make sure everything is in order and then says rather quickly, "But Judy died in 1975—cancer—which was *very* stressful. We'd been married about twenty-one years." His thoughts come out now in small, tight bunches. "We would probably still be married," he says. "That's the kind of school we're from. She got ill about '73 or '74. It was stressful, it bothered me. She passed away in 1975. For my youngsters it was traumatic. They were in their early twenties."

Jack has never linked his wife's death with his heart attack. "No," he says definitively, "because I was getting those pains before that. I retired in '75, after Judy passed away. I said, 'What the hell. There's no reason to work.' We were closing the brokerage office in Beverly Hills and we were going to move it to Century City. Instead, I just retired."

Pressing further, I suggested that his wife's death must have left a large gap in his life. "Yes," he replies, "oh sure . . . but the support was there. Our friends were very supportive. I myself was the one who ran away." He pauses and I wait for him to continue. His last thought stops him. "Why did I run away?" he asks; the question is to himself. "I don't know. I was doing nothing. But in doing nothing I was more tired. It was lousy."

There's a brief silence, one with barbs around the edges. I ask if he is angry about his wife's death.

Jack shakes his head no, but then he ponders the possibility further. "I don't know," he starts. "I've gone through analysis. We've talked about it. But . . . I don't think it was anger." Another pause follows softly, then he says assuredly, "No, there wasn't really anger. Judy and I had discussed it during the weeks before she passed away.

She had told the kids that we were a unit and there'd be some changes. But all-in-all, it was a good life. We really did have a good life." Another small silence hangs in the air. Neither of us says anything because there doesn't seem to be much to say. Slowly Jack continues the story, punctuating it occasionally with hints of remembered sadness, subtle and barely discernible. His usually even voice is softer, more thoughtful. "She died right before her fiftieth birthday," he explains. "So I say there was stress or whatever it was, but no anger. You know, sometimes people ask themselves, 'What could I have done?' But I really don't feel that way. I'm a fatalist in that respect."

Reacting to Jack's quiet rendering of his wife's death, I suggest to him that life must have seemed empty. But he bounces back with a different opinion. "You know," he contends, "there is no such thing as empty. I didn't have that feeling." He elaborates. "I hate to be alone; I must have companionship. That's one thing I saw—that this was necessary. And that's how Edie and I got together. Although we had lived within a couple of blocks of each other for twenty-some years, I never really knew Edie. I did know her husband very well though, and I can say there was no difference in the way her kids were raised or anything. Mine turned out real well and hers too, basically. Her husband, Ben, was forty-two or so when he died, and her kids were at a more impressionable age—ten, eleven. It's hard for the youngsters.

"My wife was smart. Matter of fact Edie's husband used to call my wife, Judy, the smartest gal he ever knew. Everybody said that of her. If she could handle me . . . she had to be." Jack stops to take a phone call. One call stretches into two. He looks at me sheepishly and then buzzes his secretary to hold his calls for a while.

"Judy told all her girlfriends," he remembers, " 'Give Jack about a year off and then put him and Edie together.' " He grins reflectively and he explains, "She was a pretty sharp cookie, my wife." The fond memory passes in exchange for the present. "Edie was someone whose investments I was managing after her husband had died. He was very close to me," he repeats.

Before his wife died, Jack and Judy had discussed decreasing his workload. They agreed that they were satisfied with their standard of living and decided that Jack would phase out some of his activities and establish investments satisfactory for them to maintain their life-style. After his wife's death, Jack carried out the plan and literally retired. He sold his businesses, paid off his debts and began traveling. He and Edie became a couple, traveling together, picking up remnants of lives scarred by tragedy. Throughout this time, however, he continued to experience the discomfort in his chest—and continued to ignore it, although he admits that his doctor's persistent advice to him was, 'Hey, buster, relax. Take it easy.' Ignoring this advice, he eventually found himself in the emergency room of Kaiser Permanente Clinic. And as thousands of cardiac patients before him, Jack endured the customary stay in the hospital after his heart attack and went home to recuperate, strengthen himself and consider the bypass surgery that had been recommended. I ask him what he did during that time.

"I just stayed home," he says. "I walked, exercised; I wasn't running that much, just walking around the block. Eating. I read. I'm a good reader, an avid reader. I walked, tried to strengthen myself." He thinks a minute more and adds, "I just did what I had to do to keep out of mischief. I met all the womenfolk in the apartment building, did the laundry, cleaned the house. I didn't mind doing it." In answer to my next question, he says, "No, I wasn't doing anything creative."

Depending on his mood on the particular day that you ask about his recuperation from the heart attack, Jack's response will either be jovial—as if he truly enjoyed swapping stories with the women in the laundromat—or depressed and resigned, resentful of the turn of events. The first day I spoke with him about his recuperation period, he described it as a morose, unproductive time that he resented. On the second occasion we discussed it, he pictured it as more of a happy-go-lucky lying-in period, during which there were restrictions of his activities, but understood and accepted. This vacillation is probably more a reflection of Jack's tendency not to dwell long on negatives—a predilection to pick up the loose ends and get on with things—than a symptom of emotional capriciousness.

Not long after he was released from the hospital to recuperate at home, Jack Rutta suffered a blood clot—an embolism. A clot lodged in the arteries of the heart can trigger a heart attack, but Jack was relatively fortunate; the clot, it was determined, had lodged in his lung. Although undaunted by his heart attack, Jack admits that the embolism scared him. "I didn't like that," he says, as he goes on to describe how he felt, with considerably more emotion and detail than when recounting his heart attack experience. "I had the cold sweats," he remembers, "and I was completely weak. I couldn't do anything, couldn't even yell out. The body wouldn't function. I just couldn't move," he reveals softly.

I asked if he felt he might die. "No, no," he responds impatiently. "But I didn't have control. That annoyed the hell out of me. I got real angry with this Edie of mine because she was with her son in another room when it happened. It must have been two hours that she never once came into the room I was in to check on me. I had a big beef with her on that. Finally,'' he says icily, ''she came in to check on me and she called the ambulance and they took me right into the hospital.''

I wanted to know whether he was concerned about having another heart attack. ''No,'' Jack answers. ''I knew something was wrong, but it was a completely different sensation altogether; I knew it wasn't a heart attack.''

After another brief stay in the hospital, Jack was back at home with his laundry and his books and his thoughts about bypass surgery. I asked him if he worried about having another heart attack during his recuperation time, a common, although not often expressed, concern for many heart patients. ''Fear never entered in there,'' he maintains. ''I'm almost sure that consciously or subconsciously I never had that fear.''

Something like fear or apprehension did enter Jack's mind, however, years before. Plagued by the discomfort in his chest, he decided he needed to implement some action to head off the inevitable result of a suspected heart condition.

He tilts his head back, rolls his eyes deep into his head, as if trying to count the years. ''It was in '76,'' he begins, ''when I made up my mind that something was really wrong. It was when I was in Vermont or somewhere. We had just come back from Europe. Edie and I were walking some hilly country or something and I got that hot feeling—too much to ignore. And that's when I bought the Pritikin book and started the program.

''I knew it had something to do with my heart,'' he continues. ''There was no doubt about it. That was it. And then for the next two or three years I never ate eggs; I cut out the lobster and the shrimp and the obvious things. I almost always ordered chicken, and I wouldn't order the cream sauces. Always the fish without sauce. I never have been a salt user to speak of, so I didn't tell them not to use salt, but I never added any. That became my normal eating,'' he says in his predictably practical and unselfconscious manner. ''That was no trouble. I carried that big old book around everywhere.''

Mindful that a common coping strategy of heart disease is denial, I asked Jack what made him implement such a drastic program based solely on his own speculation. Did he really know then that he was facing problems with his heart?

He ponders the question a moment. ''Did I know?'' he asks. ''Not really. I didn't know. But I knew something was going to happen. I have a very strong philosophy, which is based on the fact that the guy in the mirror can't be conned; don't try to kid him. And I really stick to that. I'm very sincere about that. I think I have good ethics, good morals; I think I have good judgment. And I'm a stubborn son-of-a-gun. Oh, when I make up my mind, it's got to be done.

"I picked Pritikin because I kept hearing about it. I'm always listening. Before that it was Adele Davis. I was always reading books on nutrition. I knew food—that's it. That's what makes you." Asked about the reaction of people around him to his new way of eating, Jack says his friends supported him in the Pritikin diet. "They all went along with it," he recalls. "Our friends respected my judgment. So if I went on chicken, they all went on chicken."

Jack describes himself as having been a "good eater—always a balanced diet. Never anything to excess. But," he concedes, "I was eating the full American diet. Lots of steak, not much fish and chicken, like I am now. But I'm not a dessert eater. No ice cream. Just a three-meal man. Steaks two or three times a week. Chicken on Fridays.

"As a kid I was a hell of an athlete. A damn good athlete. And I knew it was because of my strength, even though I was small. I was proud of my ability. I knew you had to eat. You had to have your oatmeal, your big breakfast in the morning. Outside of a little wine, drinking in moderation at all times. I've never really been drunk."

Speaking from his knowledge of a low-cholesterol, low-fat diet, Jack continues to describe the preferences of his "American" way of eating. "Eggs, now that's another story—two, three a day, raw. I loved them. I'd just drop them in the water for a minute, no more. Those eggs I love to this day. Instead of chasing twenty-year-old girls my idea of fun was to get good eggs. That's the only thing that bothered me," he admits with a sigh. "And I gave up milk. I love milk to this day. I still drink a gallon to gallon-and-a-half of milk a week—but now it's nonfat milk.

"I drank very little coffee, but I smoked, like a couple of packs a day. I quit smoking in 1971. I inhaled a cigarette wrong," he explains. "I remember I was on Venice Boulevard near La Cienega. I just started coughing, wheezing, crying. I really had tears in my eyes. So I took the pack and threw it out the window and that was it. Just like that. By then I had been having that hot esophagus and that probably had a little to do with it—stopping like that."

So like millions of Americans each year, Jack Rutta suffered a heart attack—"a coronary" as it is sometimes called; in medical terms, a myocardial infarction. And like millions of others, Jack's heart attack was a result of coronary artery disease—one or more of the arteries supplying blood to his heart had been blocked, either by a blood clot or by a large-sized plaque inhibiting the flow of the blood in the artery. Although most of us may think of the heart as a pump whose essential function is to send blood throughout the body, the human heart is itself a muscle and like all muscles, needs its share of oxygen and nutrients. If for some reason the flow of blood is cut off to an area of the heart, the muscle cells in that area may die of oxygen and nutrient starvation. Although other muscles may continue to survive without oxygen, in approximately twenty minutes the cells of an oxygen-starved heart begin to die. This is what accounts for the damage caused by a heart attack.

To more thoroughly understand the physiology of this process, a closer look at the biology of an artery is required. The central part of the artery through which the blood flows is called the lumen. The coronary arteries lie on the surface of the heart, so unlike other arteries in the body, they aren't buried or protected by a layer of muscle or supporting tissue. Almost as soon as we're born, the lining of the lumen is subject to small injuries that leave tiny nicks or scars in this interior artery wall. Repair is accomplished as muscle cells enter the area and multiply. Unfortunately those injured areas serve later as the focal point for the development of obstructions that may eventually close the artery, obstructions referred to as plaques. All plaques start as muscle repair cells. Depending on a number of factors, these scarlike masses contain cholesterol, fat and some calcium. If a plaque grows large enough, it may block the artery itself, or it may become the nucleus around which a blood clot will grow, or it may cause what is called a vascular spasm. In any event, the result is the same—interference in blood flow.

At the time of his heart attack, Jack was apparently suffering from this kind of plaque buildup. The particular danger of coronary artery disease is that it is usually symptomless until it advances to the stage where the individual is subject to serious interference in coronary blood supply and thus a heart attack.

The arterial deposits that may eventually threaten to close off blood flow contain primarily fat and cholesterol. Cholesterol itself is a fatlike, pearly substance found in all animal fats and oils, in bile, blood and brain tissue, in the liver, kidney and adrenal glands. A certain amount of cholesterol is essential to maintain bodily functions, primarily to produce certain essential hormones and to help build cells. The human body manufactures approximately 1,000 milligrams of cholesterol a day. However, excess serum cholesterol—the amount of cholesterol circulating in a person's blood—has long been suspected as a contributing factor in the development of plaque. This plaque in turn can lead to obstruction or narrowing of the arteries, a condition that in its advanced form is designated atherosclerosis.

Cholesterol is found in a great variety of the foods we eat— notably eggs, dairy products, meat and fish. Ingestion of foods containing large amounts of cholesterol and saturated fat from animal sources contributes to the buildup of cholesterol in the blood, which in turn is deposited in the lining of the veins and arteries. Although controversy continues as to the exact equation between cholesterol and heart disease, it is generally considered advisable to reduce the intake of dietary cholesterol and fat. Likewise cigarettes, excessive alcohol and caffeine intake have been implicated as risk factors in heart disease. (Recently, researchers have identified two types of cholesterol—HDL and LDL, abbreviations for high density lipoprotein (blood fat) and low density lipoprotein. The LDLs are the repositories for dietary cholesterol, while the HDLs actually function as fat-collectors, sweeping the loose cholesterol into the liver, from which it is expelled from the body.)

In many unfortunate ways, Jack Rutta's case was typical. There had been no heart disease in his immediate family. "Pappy," he says, "went to eighty and then died of a stroke. Strong as they come. My mother lived into her eighties; my grandfather till over a hundred. All my uncles lived to the eighties. The longevity was there." Given that kind of heredity and few overt symptoms, Jack had little reason to suspect heart disease in himself.

But typical in many ways, Jack was an anomaly in others. With hard work and initiative Jack had amassed enough wealth to make his family comfortable and to enhance their status. And having accumulated all of this, he relinquished it at an age when most people would be settling in to savor it. It's difficult to speculate what would have happened had Jack's wife lived and they had been able to live the quieter life they planned. What did happen, however, was something quite different.

II

"You can't kid that guy in the mirror."

I asked Jack if he thought one of the reasons he experienced his heart attack even after he'd endorsed the Pritikin Program was because he hadn't started to change his life-style soon enough.

He rocks back and forth in the soft secretarial chair, thinks for a moment and then says flatly, "No, I'm a Type A individual. I hold it within me and I'm hyper. That's why I had it. I had atherosclerosis and one has to feed on the other."

Today the concept of the Type A peronality has become part of the popular wisdom among heart patients, some of whom appear to claim the label as a badge of identification—or perhaps an excuse for what's happened to them. Heart patients often seize upon Type A behavior, which is a function of a particular personality, as a way of relegating the cause of their difficulties to factors outside their control. In fact, a 1980 government study, undertaken with a select group of medical centers, clearly identified the Type A personality as a risk factor in the development of heart disease. However, in 1973, when the concept was first introduced by Doctors Meyer Friedman and Ray Rosenman, it represented a radical departure from conventional thinking about cardiac diagnosis and rehabilitation. And if Dr. Friedman has not yet succeeded in convincing the medical establishment that the ramifications of this personality type is a fundamental cause of heart disease, his theory and research have shed light on behavior patterns that seem synonymous with its incidence.

The Type A behavior pattern most associated with heart disease—and both Jack Rutta and Fred Rizk acknowledge this as a major contributing factor in their own illness—is a chronic sense of "time urgency" coupled with an excessively competitive drive. In other words, trying to do too much in too little time. Another aspect of the pattern is a sense of easily aroused, generalized hostility. Seeking to accomplish more and more in less and less time and unable to do so, the Type A individual develops a sense of unfocused anger and frustration. Friedman and his associates are not describing a psychosis or a "complex of worries or phobias" or even an obsession, but a socially acceptable, indeed, often praised, "form of conflict." In point of fact, the socially condoned Type A can claim kinship with elements of the Puritan work ethic, our all-American belief in the value of hard work and accomplishment.

Time is the enemy of the Type A. Even if his time were increased or expanded, he would quickly fill it with additional challenges. According to Friedman, the "fundamental sickness of the Type A personality is his peculiar failure to accept the undeniable fact that a man's time *can* be exhausted by his activities."

Why should a person strive to expand time until it finally implodes upon itself? Because that person has lost or perhaps never developed an intrinsic means of measuring his own fundamental worth, instead utilizing the yardstick of numbers of achievements, which must come at an ever-accelerating rate. The Type A's methods often backfire, however, causing further insecurity instead of the status and acceptance he seeks. The haste with which he pursues accomplishment forces him to constantly measure his achievements against an ever more rapidly changing group of peers and superiors. Charged with accumulating maximum achievement in nominal time, this individual must forever match himself against new criteria of success. Additionally and perhaps most importantly for Type As facing the aftereffects of a heart attack or reckoning with the realities of heart disease, the unavoidable result of more and more and faster and faster is loss of the ability to think creatively. To save time, the Type A is forced to act in a stereotypical manner, regardless of whether or not this is applicable to his new challenges.

Without creative thoughts, or keenness of judgment, the Type A substitutes speed. If there is continuity in his milieu and its demands remain fundamentally unchanged, he will appear to retain the capability for the "brilliant moves" he has become known for. Once beyond the familiar, however, and bereft of adaptability, he risks failure and collapse. Many Type As confront their physical limits before hitting this psychological wall.

Freidman concludes that conversion from Type A to what he considers the more even and adaptable Type B may reduce the chances of heart attack by half. Although many of the men and women who woefully, or proudly, lay claim to "being Type A" may not fully understand Friedman's theory or its implications, they tend to identify strongly with the condition of always attempting to do too much and never being satisfied. Another component of Type A behavior is a predilection to be involved in the lives of others while being unable to ask for or accept aid or advice for oneself. Although Type As may intuit that this pattern can only produce adverse affects, without help, they are usually at a loss as to how strategies of reform might be implemented.

And so it is that Jack so easily implicates his Type A behavior in the development of his illness. Mindful of the usual pattern of coronary artery disease, I asked him if he had had any symptoms right before his attack. "No," he answers, "it was the same thing. Always the same thing—the hot esophagus—that funny feeling. A little more frequently that's all. I knew it, because I really wasn't doing anything physical. And there was a little more stress. I could feel the stress. It wasn't work stress," he explains, "because there was no work. I was doing nothing." When I asked what kind of stress he thought it was, Jack responds, "I can't answer that. I just knew that something was bothering me and I know there was something there. That's why then I was really Spartan."

The issue of control, an essential element in the Type A personality, appears repeatedly in Jack's speech. Pressed to superhuman efforts, the Type A attempts to keep all his balls in the air and bouncing by regulating even the most trivial aspects of his life and work. Delegation is difficult because it means relinquishing some portion of this control to another person or persons. Jack Rutta recognizes this desire for control as fundamental to his character. It is also an issue that rings familiar among other heart patients. I asked Jack if he ever tried to loosen some of his need to control people and things.

"Yes," he says languidly, slowly sidling up to the subject. "I work at it. I'm letting go a little bit; I'm deliberately doing it. But I like the shelves to be neat, the refrigerator organized—it's the engineer mentality. I'm more fastidious than the normal person. I know exactly where things are at any time."

I reflect that this takes a lot of energy. "I know that," he acknowledges, "but that's me. I know I can do it right, but I also know you have to delegate authority. And I like doing that . . . if," he adds slyly, "there's enough for me to do." He sits back and thinks for a minute. His secretary comes over to give him a message. They confer and he slowly turns back to me, ready to issue one of his kiddingly serious observations. "Do you realize," he asks, "that the average person doesn't delegate authority because there isn't enough for him to do? I found that out. I can do three jobs at the same time. But people like that fear they might get lost in the shuffle and not be needed."

It's an interesting thought. I asked Jack if he knows that fear. Without missing a beat, he says, "I know that I'm the greatest."

"At what?" I asked.

"At just about everything."

I decide to continue the bantering. "Did it take a while to get to that, or did you always know it?"

"You mean," he grins, "was I always humble?" I laugh and he continues. "I think I knew from the beginning. I've always been able to do it. I got no support from my family, no love. Nothing. Would you believe that? I grew up too early, maybe. I really missed out on childhood, there's no doubt about that. But I played every sport. I was one of those high school phenomenons.

"My father wasn't interested in my sports accomplishments, not at all. 'Go make money,' he said. I was making more money than he was and I was just working part-time. I always had something going." He seems comfortable with that thought. " 'What makes Sammy run . . .' " he says and then out of the blue, "and that's deceptive because I appear relaxed all the time."

I agree with him that he always appears very loose. "That's what's amazing," he says. "I think I'm relaxed right now." I confirm that he looks relaxed.

"That's what I'm saying," he repeats. "That's very deceptive. But I've always said there isn't a problem I can't solve, I don't care what it is. And the ego trips—they're gone, they went away. One day, I got very smart. I paid off all the debt I owed. I'd always set goals and always attained them."

Obviously Jack Rutta is a man with a mind of his own and it is infinitely practical. As he talks cautiously about his bouts with therapy, it appears to be an important matter to him that he cool down his Type A inclinations. I asked if in his therapy, he'd been introduced to the concept of getting in touch with the child within himself. He relates to the question immediately. "Yes. This is the dichotomy in there. The child, I can bring him out. I went through all of this with Edie. It was very important. I hope it helped. But then the adult comes back, and the adult makes things serious." Jack looks frustrated with that remark, but I empathize easily with what he says. The over-responsible adult can be merciless in its need for accomplishment and control.

When I asked if he had any second thoughts about bypass surgery, Jack shot back, "I wanted to do it. Number one, I had read the book—*Physician Heal Thyself*—just before that I had read about Type A and B. It looked to me that bypasses made sense, so I wasn't against the bypass, no way. But it was the old story with me: 'If you'll let me perform the bypass myself, I'll go in'—no argument with that." He laughs at the impossibility of that happening and adds, "My doctor told me, though, 'I'll let you look up to the last minute.' "

"I really wanted to do things right," he continues lightly. "Like I insisted on meeting the anesthesiologist before the operation. They asked me, 'What for?' I said, 'He's the guy who's going to put me under with those machines. I want to see him first.' "

The com line on Jack's phone rings. He hesitates a second, reaches for the phone and steals a sidelong glance at me. A brief moment of indecision. He opts for the phone. The conversation, with an old friend about a proposed stock transaction, is brief. Jack hangs up and reminds his secretary to hold his calls.

So Jack Rutta accepted the idea of a coronary bypass but wanted to control it as far as he could. "Yep," he chuckles, with the same kind of self-mocking humor Jim Irwin turns in on himself, "just in case something changed and I didn't have to have it. I always ask myself with something like that, 'Is it necessary?' "

"What convinced you it was?" I asked.

"I made the decision. I was doing nothing. No sex. Nothing was going on. So I knew something was wrong. And I knew it had to be done. I was just hanging around the house. I wasn't conscious of any emotional reaction, but I'm the kind of guy who puts that kind of thing aside.'' This is dangerous territory, and he moves the subject quickly forward. ''Turned out,'' he says, ''they only did a triple bypass. They were going to do four, but the day before surgery, the doctor brought in somebody else to examine me. There were three vessels blocked. One was eighty percent, the smallest one forty percent and the other one was seventy percent blocked. I have a drawing of it. The doctor gave it to me because I was asking a lot of questions.

''I watched him doing the angiogram. I remember at one point he said to me, 'We're coming to it. See where it's harder to go through. That's our problem area—eighty percent blockage.' I saw it,'' Jack says matter-of-factly.

The angiogram that Jack and other cardiac patients speak of is a diagnostic tool used to determine if there is narrowing or closing in one or more of the heart's three major arteries or their branches. A catheter is fed through an artery, usually in the groin area, until it reaches the arteries of the heart. Radiopaque material is inserted through the catheter separately into each artery and a series of X rays are rapidly taken. A highly sensitive technique, its early use was marred by the real apprehension that it might actually trigger a heart attack in some people. Since its development during the '60s, however, the technique and instrumentation—assisted by computers—have become more sophisticated and the danger of experiencing a heart attack during the procedure has been almost completely eliminated.

I wanted to know how Jack felt watching the doctor examine the arteries of his heart. ''I was inquisitive,'' he remembers. ''I wasn't angry. I was just happy that there was an option—a way to get out of it. I'm the luckiest guy alive. I look at the bypass scars and everything—that doesn't bother me.'' He lifts up the left pant leg of his well-tailored suit to show me. ''A Japanese guy did the cutting on the leg,'' he says. ''Different guy did up here,'' he points to his chest. ''I didn't realize that one person didn't do the whole thing. A guy named Mendeze did the top side. Jerry did the heart.'' He repeats it again, ''Eighty-seventy-forty.''

''Do you think you were lucky you had the heart attack when you did?''

''Yep,'' he answers without hesitation. ''I didn't want to be cut open. I wanted to see if there was a way around it. Because,'' he grins, ''I knew they weren't going to let me do the operating. But when it came time and there was nothing else to do, I went. It seems to me that your body's such a wonderful thing, why resent something that can help it?'' Then he adds philosophically, ''And there's always tomorrow.''

So, like thousands of other Americans, Jack Rutta opted for bypass surgery. But unlike many people, he stuck to the diet he had implemented before the heart attack and before the surgery. Unfortunately many people feel so good after having a bypass procedure they neglect to remember what caused their problem in the first place. In fact there is evidence to suggest that in the first few weeks after bypass surgery, the transplanted veins, smaller than the arteries whose function they replace, thicken in order to handle the higher pressure of arterial blood, and at this stage they are particularly susceptible to deposits of cholesterol that can clog their interior and inhibit their ability to handle blood flow.

Worse news comes from the Montreal Heart Institute, where a 1981 study found that after ten years, eighty percent of the original arteries and the grafted veins of patients who had undergone bypass surgery had become diseased. And the coronary unit of Mount Sinai Hospital in New York City reports that repeat bypasses are on the rise. William Castelli, medical director of the ongoing Framingham Heart Study in Framingham, Massachusetts, which has monitored the city's population for heart disease since the '40s, warns against possible artery thickening aftereffects of bypass surgery. Castelli maintains that reverting to the former high-risk life-style is, in effect, a decision to close down what is left of the original arteries as well as the new bypass veins.

Having changed his diet before the heart attack, Jack had one leg up on the problems that often confront bypass patients—where to go from there. He continued his dietary program and gradually got back into exercise.

After his heart attack, his doctor had placed him on Inderal and prescribed nitroglycerin for his angina. Inderal, a medication that belongs to a general class of drugs called beta blockers, is the second most prescribed drug in this country. It is used primarily for individuals who have recently suffered a heart attack, and for people with high blood pressure. The beta blockers, introduced in 1966, block nervous impulses to the heart, so that in moments of physical or emotional stress, when the pulse begins to quicken and increases the demand on the heart, the beta blocker actually works to lower the heart rate, reducing the need for oxygen. The beta blockers were welcomed by medical science as the first drug with the potential capability of prolonging survival in patients with coronary artery disease. They are part of the estimated $3.5 billion annual market for cardiovascular medications.

"One of the first things I wanted to do," says Jack, "was to get off medication as fast as possible. That was my goal. Aspirin to me is a medication. It took well over a year and we did it by stages. My doctor was testing me all along. Inderal was the one that took me a long time to get off."

When I suggested that some people continue to carry nitroglycerin with them, even after they have had bypass surgery, Jack responds confidently, "Not me. The only thing I still have is some Valium. A bottle of Valium, one hundred Valium will last me about three years. Matter of fact I buy the five-milligram size and break them in half. Took one the other day—I was feeling tight."

Asked what advice he'd have for someone who is trying to change their diet and life-style, he says immediately, "Ask yourself," he begins, initiating a dialogue with an imaginary stranger, 'What do you need it for? What's good about it? Tastes good? Great—there are other things you can satisfy the taste with. But the thing is it isn't good for you, so let's get away from it. You don't have to miss it, so don't miss it. Yes, I'd love to have a—whatever it is—but I'm not supposed to have it, so that's it.' It makes sense," he concludes. "When you can truthfully say something and believe it, it's easy. I'm not trying to convince myself.

"Take an example—a friend of mine went to St. Vincent's and had an angiogram and bypasses. He looks terrible. I told him, 'You're doing something wrong.' He's not following the diet. He's a refugee—he was in the camps and all that. I guess there's something I don't know. When he was first going through it, I loaned him the Pritikin book. I told him what to do. But he's not doing it."

"How do you find eating like this?" I asked him.

"It's boooorrring," he drawls.

"How do you stay with it if it's boring?"

"I do it; that's all. I do it. I know I should be doing it and that's it. I'm stubborn. You've got to remember that the basic personality is very stubborn. Whatever I make up my mind to do, I do. I can't be tempted. I don't have any little routines in terms of cheating. I don't say, 'Tonight I'm going to do it.' I just follow through with what I'm supposed to do. We're out with a group—like Sunday night I went to the Philharmonic. We ate at the Hungry Tiger downtown and I had chicken. They know me pretty well and the people we were with. The waiter comes out and says, 'Jack, there is some lovely salmon'—every now and then they have a decent chef down there, believe it or not—'it's gorgeous.' He's not conning me, I know. 'With a lovely cream sauce.' And I say to him, 'Chicken, that's it.' And a couple of glasses of wine. I can put lemon juice on the salad or have it dry. I eat my bread dry. I love the taste of French bread, so why put butter on it? That's what I did before even.

"I like a nice gooey piece of sweets," he admits, "and if I see it, I might have it now and then, but if I'm going to have a sweet dessert, I make sure it's a Spartan meal. I don't ever have dessert if I've had a big meal. As a matter of fact I love to eat before six o'clock. I want the meal digested before I go to bed."

Warming to the subject, he continues, "We play a lot of bridge. I will play bridge and not have anything. So the people know already that I don't give a damn what they're serving. Always the new people feel insulted, because they've got the little candies and whatever they set out for bridge, all these nuts, cheese. I don't touch it. I'll sit down afterward and I'll take a decaf, and to people who know me real well, I'll say, 'Give me skinny milk.' They just bring out a glass of milk and I can take that with whatever they've got. My close friends will always have angel food cake—no egg yolks in that. In somebody's house," he says with a shrug, "I just sit down and try to be as quiet as possible, unobtrusive."

He cracks one of his small captivating smiles. "The joke," he says, "is that Jack has his cookie and milk every evening. Now I have angel food cake instead of my cookies, which might have been an Oreo-type cookie. Every morning I have the roughage, you know, bran. No sugar, salt, anything in it. Big bowl every morning with banana and juice.

"Hey," he says, nuzzling another thought forward, "I love Mexican food. I will go and eat rice cooked with chicken or I eat plain chicken. There's no harm in that. Or a chicken tostada. I stay away from the beans because they cook them in the lard. The rice they don't touch. There are a couple of places I found that make this chicken and rice with vegetables. That's not bad. I could probably eat that every day and it wouldn't hurt me. And I have a Chinese place that I go to. They don't fry anything. I don't buy fried.

"Then I've got an Italian restaurant," he continues. "There I have rolled chicken with some herbs, nice sauce over it, but it's not too bad. And I like pasta. I'm going to China for almost a month. I'll tell them I'm a vegetarian. It's the same thing when I go on an airplane. In Mexico, I try to get fish whenever I can. The dramatic changes to me were skinny milk and eggs. I do miss the eggs. I can tell you right now, a good cheese and egg omelet would be wonderful."

Remembering other people's comments about adherence, I asked

Jack what he feels is the worst part of eating like this. He fires back, "There's no worst part. I just don't desire.

"I'm never fighting a craving because . . ." He stops himself, bounces back with the notion he's looking for. "It's discipline," he says. "I'm too damned disciplined. That might be a drawback too. Being stubborn, I can regulate or control it easily. If I'm not supposed to have it, that's it. We were in Lake Tahoe on Labor Day and we went upstairs to the top of the Wagon Wheel. That night they were featuring lobster. The rest of them ordered the special. I told the waiter, 'Bring me some swordfish and a potato and string beans.' He kept looking at me. 'That's it,' I said. Afterward he came back in and brought the dessert table and they all had desserts. That doesn't bother me, not one bit."

"What if you do eat something like the prime rib you had the other night," I asked. "Do you feel bad about it?"

He laughs widely. "I enjoy it. Maybe that helps me stay on it the rest of the time—I'm in control again. Maybe that's the feature, I'm in control. I want it. I can have it. I wonder if it isn't because of rigidity," he muses. "Whatever you want to call it. I'm one of these guys who, if we had a chocolate fair, could walk though it and never taste anything. I don't think it really bothers me, in the sense of wanting to do it. How's that? I'm not conscious of fighting it. They say to me, 'Try, try. Try this; try that.' My response is, 'What do I want to try it for? Yes, it smells wonderful and looks beautiful.' "

Because he decided to reform his life-style before the heart attack and before the bypass, Jack implies that he doesn't need to fall back on memories of those events to keep him on track. "No, that's been decided long ago," he says. "That's it. I'm not consciously aware of it. I do have a very conscious sense of control—a wonderful thing. Sure it puts stress on me. I know that—like giving up smoking, for the first few weeks, but I did it. I said, 'The hell with it, I don't need that.' And I tell you honestly I still would like to smoke but I don't. I'm strong. I know that it has to be something that I'm doing, because it isn't a fear." He pauses a moment and then he says, "You've got to be oxnow. Do you know what that is?" When I shake my head no, he explains. "Oxnow is greater than stubborn," he says proudly. I laugh and ask him if that works for him in business.

"Objectivity, not emotions," he answers. "I try to stay away from the emotions."

"Maybe a craving for something is emotion."

"Yes, I believe so," he agrees.

"And the control is intellectual?"

"And that could be building up to the A type of individual I would imagine,'' he says but lets the thought slide, uninclined to investigate it further.

The workday is drawing to a close. It's time for Jack to head home to dinner. More likely he will be heading to a Philharmonic concert, or a Lakers basketball game. Or maybe it's his night for his Bible group, or maybe his Brandeis University sponsored study group is meeting. Or maybe tonight's the night for square dancing. "I gave up my Ram tickets," he tells me. "It seemed like we were going out fourteen nights a week. What'd you need that for?" he asks rhetorically. When I asked about his taste in music, Jack explains to me that he goes to special Philharmonic concerts on Friday nights because there is a preconcert lecture.

Jack Rutta returned to work in 1982, two years after his bypass surgery, as he says, "to see what it was all about after the heart attack." He maintains he likes what he's doing and isn't pressed right now to discover something else.

"I work with some retarded children. I go to the Brandeis group to partake of whatever they can offer me. Self-gratification is the most important thing now, but it has to be intellectual. I'll have to fall over something now—a big challenge. I won't aggressively go out and find it. For what purpose?" he asks. "See, that's the thing. There are definite motivating forces—dollars and ego are the two I'm aware of."

"What about self-satisfaction?" I wondered.

"No," he answers. "That's in there under ego. Self-gratification? That's a subchapter. I don't want to invent the wheel; I don't want to pioneer or proselytize. I'm always curious, that's the self-gratification part of it. The satisfaction is there—it's been done. I really don't know of anything out there that I really should be doing. Maybe that's why I have satisfaction."

We talked for a few moments about friends who have conquered illness and others who haven't been lucky. Jack relates to the survivors. "I would never give up," he contends. "I think if it was inevitable, I would pass and say, 'Let's call it quits'—if I knew this was a terminal something. But right now, everything's great, tomorrow will be coming. But," he adds, speaking slowly, "if I don't have control of my functions or myself I don't think I'd want to continue." He grins and laughs, "I really want to be the boss." He pauses and says slyly, "I guess that's it."

"What's good about being the boss?"

"I can go and do what I want," he answers. "That's what being the boss means. It's a good feeling. However, I don't mind people telling me what to do. As I said, I'm not going to be the innovator. I'm not going to invent the wheel. But I will help perfect it. I think that's the difference.

"My ego has been satiated," he concludes easily. "The ego has been taken care of."

As Jack speaks, an older man, probably in his seventies, approaches the counter in front of us and signals to Jack, who waves to him. The gentleman says meekly that he'd like Jack's advice about an investment. Jack jumps up, excuses himself, walks over and shakes hands with the old man, who pulls a wrinkled envelope out of the pocket of his well-pressed and brushed sport coat. Jack looks carefully at the material the man digs from the envelope. In a moment, he has assessed his client's problem and assures him that he has nothing to worry about. He pats the old man on the shoulder, shakes his hand again and sends him on his way. He comes back and perches himself on the small chair.

"You kind of have to reassure people like that. That's part of my job." He waits a minute and then for effect says, "Actually I have a harem." He holds off another minute for my reaction. I laugh; he continues. "My harem consists of thirteen women who have outlived their menfolks. Wealthy women. I have three answering machines in the house for them. They call me with all kinds of questions—from what color am I going to paint this or that, to whether they're getting the best price on a painting or a new car. Whatever it is, they call me up. I say, 'Talk to the machine and I'll get back to you.' And I always do. I don't charge them a nickel. I just feel obligated to a bunch of people who were nice to me for many years."

"That's very nice of you."

"No, no," he counters. "I'm selfish. I'll tell you why. Because I mess around with some retarded children. I donate a day a week every other week working with a youngster. The organization's called Goal; it's in Beverly Hills. So these gals, when I need anything, write the checks. That's fair enough. And it's really nothing. They all have so much money that I don't give it a second thought. No matter where I hide it or put it, it's there and they can't spend it. Luckily I think every one of them will donate their money to various charities."

He goes back to his original thought. "Maybe it's because I can look in the mirror and be happy. You can't kid that guy in the mirror. You can never fool him.

"And, you know what?" he asks. And not waiting for an answer he says, "He ain't too bad a guy at all."

Chapter 4

Fred Rizk, 60, president of Rizk Construction Company, Houston. Married; one son, 26, another, six months.

Diagnosis: angina pectoris, symptomatic of coronary artery disease; bypass surgery recommended.

I

"I didn't figure I'd be a man with bypasses in me."

Fred Rizk came in the backdoor of his townhouse not far from the Houston Galleria at about four o'clock in the afternoon. His wife, Sylvia, and I had been drinking iced tea at the kitchen table and catching up on news. Fred was hungry, and he had no intention of eating alone. He ransacked the fridge, pulling out various dishes of Pritikin-style food that Helen, the cook, had prepared—a curried chicken and vegetables (short on the chicken), a Lebanese lentil dish served with nonfat yogurt and homemade nonfat yogurt cheese, Syrian bread, a variation of Pritikin bread Fred had discovered somewhere, and more iced tea. As he ate, Fred asked for comments on the food, established my itinerary for the next five days and described the slight nuances in his health that had occurred since my last visit. After lunch, I proposed a walk. Fred recommended a nap. I took the nap. It turned out I needed it for the days ahead.

Later—at eight o'clock on a hot Texas Saturday night—Fred and I climbed into Sylvia's air-conditioned Mercedes and headed for the Houstonian, the exclusive health club where Fred works out. It was early in the summer, so the sky was still very light and the air muggy and hot. At the club, I was assigned a locker and agreed to meet Fred on the track. The Houstonian's indoor track runs around a core of weight-lifting machines and mirrored partitions set up for aerobic exercise. Together Fred and I looked at the clock, both seemingly ready to commit to a certain timed workout. We started around the track, talking about the value of walking versus running and about Fred's knee injury, which has slowed him from his usual jog to this slower-paced walk.

Just as I was adapting to the rhythm of our pace, however, Fred decided we should try the outdoor track that laces its way through the trees and shrubs surrounding the hotel and health club buildings. I followed him out the door and down a flight of steps to the track. The heat had begun to dissipate, although the soggy humidity still lingered. We began to walk and after the first lap around the track, Fred started to talk, introducing the subject of his illness.

I asked him when he first noticed his angina pains.

"In 1979, I believe it was," he answers. "I started having these pains in my chest. They didn't go away, so I went to the doctor. I had an old back injury, so we thought maybe the pain was related to that. They couldn't find anything, but I still had the pain. This went on for a while. Finally they decided it had to be something else. One thing they thought it might be was my heart. So they took blood and did an angiogram. My cholesterol then was in the area of 275 to 300.

"The high cholesterol wasn't the only reason they decided to do the angiogram," he continues. "I kept having these pains and nobody could figure out what they were. Even at rest I had pains. So the only way they could find out if it was my heart was through the angiogram."

I asked Fred if he had any apprehension when his doctor suggested the angiogram.

His answer is quick. "That didn't bother me," he says. "I knew I'd be OK. I knew there'd be nothing wrong with my heart, so what did I care about an angiogram? I just wanted to get it over with. I didn't even think about it in terms of danger."

Aware of Fred's impatience and preference for quick resolution of any problem that might appear in his life, I asked him what he thought about the results of the angiogram. "I didn't believe it," he replies with conviction, ". . . that I could have blocked arteries." There is a brief silence. "But *they* believed it," he adds coldly.

Questioned about whether he had any immediate emotional reaction to the diagnosis of heart disease, Fred replies quickly, "Oh, I had a lot of emotion, because I've always been very . . . explosive—and I still am." He stops, notices that he doesn't like the word explosive but decides not to spend any time on it. "Anyhow, I'm not the type that likes to feel handicapped," he says with classic understatement. "And that started years ago when I ruptured the disk in my back, which was very depressing. It was the same way with the heart problem; I couldn't believe there was something wrong with me physically. I couldn't believe it wasn't something you could overcome." Fred admits he was distressed by the possibility that he might have to alter substantially his life-style. "I had never wanted to change my life-style before when I had that ruptured disk and I felt this heart business was just another handicap."

Fred Rizk is for the most part a very private person. His wife revealed quietly to me that he is uncomfortable in the public eye and has always shunned publicity. It appears by his answers to my questions that he is also not generally accustomed to talking about himself and not totally comfortable doing so. This is not a man who has spent hours and dollars in therapy or who "burdens" his friends with his problems. His answers to my questions are brief and stated in short, simple terms, and with finality, as if this superficial rendering of the situation takes into account all possible ramifications. It's necessary to press continually harder in order to fill in the details.

I asked Fred how long it was from his first experience of chest pain until the diagnosis of heart disease was conclusive.

"From the time I first went to the doctor for the treadmill to when I went back for the angiogram," he reflects, "it was two or three months, I would imagine." He explains further, "Because of the ruptured disk—that happened maybe fifteen years ago—I had been walking to take care of my back, not aerobic-type walking, just walking. But I may have passed the treadmill because of that, because I was used to exercising. I was very regular about it. When it rained, I'd go out to the airport and walk in the tunnels."

"Even then I felt my problem was food. I ate fish maybe once a year," he says dramatically, "and only loaded with tartar sauce, and I didn't even like it then."

I smile at the disgust in his voice over fish, but it's obvious that the subject of his former unhealthy eating habits is a very serious matter to Fred. "I had meat at least three times a day," he continues. "Bacon and eggs in the morning, and pancakes; sweets three times a day. Everything fried. I hated salads. Still do.

"So," he summarizes, "it was meat and potatoes fried, and with catsup and mayonnaise. I didn't like vegetables at all. And, of course, no less than a quarter, more like a half-gallon of ice cream every night. English toffee was my favorite for six, seven years. Then pralines and cream. No chocolate," he says unswervingly, "just English toffee and pralines and cream."

Anticipating my next question, he adds, "No cigarettes, but I was smoking cigars, heavy." When I ask how heavy, he thinks a minute.

"Well, between shaving and until I went to bed, I smoked them steady, between ten and, say, fifteen cigars a day. I drank socially but not very much. I never did care for alcohol. If I had one glass of wine, I was ready to sleep. I'd start yawning." He ponders it another minute and then says, "I'm getting a taste for it now—just barely. I could enjoy it now, I think, because now anything different tastes good." We both laugh.

"And I was very heavy on caffeine," he says, then he adds, dramatically, "I ate out almost every day for thirty or thirty-three years, three meals a day. I ate very, very few meals at home."

I asked Fred if he enjoyed food.

"I like sweets," he answers. "I don't care for anything else. Back then I ate steak, because what else are you going to order when you go to a restaurant? What do they have—steak or fish—and you know what I think of fish. I also ate Italian food, spaghetti and all that, but basically I was a steak and eggs man." Then he looks at me, smiles faintly and says, "I still unconsciously look at the desserts on a menu. In fact, I always look at them first, before I order—even though I can't order any now. If I had my way, I could do without all the kinds of foods in the world but dessert. They could give me only dessert for the rest of my life and I'd be the happiest man in the world."

Fred's comments on sweets remind me of the story he once told me about trying, and failing to break the habit of eating ice cream. "I tried," he says, "but it never worked. I ate it steadily for two days, but it didn't help at all. I thought I'd get tired of it, but I still wanted the ice cream.

"So," he says as we complete another lap, wrapping up the subject of food, "when they took the angiogram, I was in reasonably good shape because I was walking, but now I know I was overloading my system with the food."

I wondered if he considered stress a factor in his life.

"There was always high stress," he answers. "Back then, I'd start working at six-thirty or seven o'clock in the morning and sometimes quit at about nine or ten o'clock at night. And that was a steady day. When we went through a crisis, I'd be working Saturdays and Sundays."

I asked if he knows why he kept such an intense pace. "That's a lot of work," I suggest to him.

He agrees. "It is a lot of work. But when you're trying to strive to get ahead . . ." His thought trails off; he finishes it unceremoniously, ". . . even though I may never use the money that I've got."

The fractured pace of questions and answers continues, seemingly keeping time with our quick-paced walking. I ask if money is important.

Without hesitation he says, "I don't think money is important at all. I think the important thing is success. The money's like a report card. I've been up and down like a yo-yo in this business. Building's a cyclical business, but I wouldn't know anything else to do. I like it. I like the excitement. It's a gamble; it's the only kind of gambling I like. I don't care for cards, dice, that kind of gambling."

The discomfort in his chest that finally brought Fred to his doctor goes by the medical name angina pectoris—a term used to describe a pain in the front and middle of the chest that tends to radiate down either arm (usually the left) or up the neck to the jaw (which is why Jack Rutta reported a soreness in his jaw when he suffered the heart attack in his car). Although the term can be applied to any discomfort in the chest area, when the pain is experienced by heart patients it is generally considered to be caused by a temporary shortage of blood to one or more areas of the heart, a scarcity blessedly short of what would trigger a heart attack. In a sense, patients who suffer angina are the lucky ones—they're notified, so to speak, of their disease and have the opportunity to take action before it blossoms into a full-scale attack. In Fred's case, however, the diagnosis of his condition was complicated by the fact that he had performed well on his treadmill test and that his pain was initially identified as a possible result of his ruptured disk.

The human heart beats busily eighty times each minute, which makes for approximately 115,000 beats each day and a little under 42,000,000 beats a year. On any given day, the heart pumps some 4,300 gallons of blood. Only five percent of that supply is allotted to nourish the heart, supplied by way of the coronary arteries. The heart muscle is divided into two sides, each with an atrium, where blood collects, and a ventricle, from which the blood is pumped out of the heart. The right atrium receives blood that has already circulated throughout the body, full of carbon dioxide, passing it to the right ventricle, which in turn pumps it into the lungs to be reoxygenated. From there it returns to the left atrium and then into the left ventricle, from which it is subsequently pumped out of the heart to all parts of the body.

The coronary arteries, through which the heart receives its supply of oxygen and nutrients, are usually but a quarter of an inch thick at their widest, in some places only one-eighth of an inch. The largest is the left coronary artery, running along the top of the heart and then dividing into two branches. The circumflex artery travels along the left edge of the heart, its branches circling the left side and onto the back. The right coronary artery serves the right side, and a branch serves the bottom of the heart. What is called the left anterior descending artery supplies the entire front wall of the heart's crucial left ventricle, its two main branches spreading across its surface and into the heart's interior. Thus it is blockage in the left main, as it's ordinarily called, that provides doctors and patients the most cause for alarm, particularly if the blockage occurs before the artery breaks into its two branches. Serious blockage before this branching almost always indicates immediate bypass surgery.

Fred Rizk's angiogram revealed a sixty percent blockage in one of the main branches of the important left anterior descending artery, as well as significant blockage in two small-to-medium-size secondary branches, estimated at eighty-five and ninety percent respectively. This meant that for Fred, the news was both bad and good. While the angiogram confirmed that he was indeed suffering from heart disease and that one branch of the left artery was involved, the other branch was completely free of blockage. Also, the degree of blockage in the involved branch was less serious than might have been indicated by Fred's experience of pain (at that time, he was reporting his incidence of angina as occurring as much as two or three times a day).

Because of these factors and because Fred had not received any prior treatment for his heart condition, his doctor chose to recommend "medical therapy"—cardiac drugs—and to hold off bypass until Fred's response to medication could be assessed. Like millions of heart patients, Fred was prescribed the old-faithful beta blocker, Inderal, along with a number of other medications, including Persantine—a vasodilator to dilate the coronary arteries and increase blood flow. He was also advised to continue his activities in moderation.

Fred Rizk is 60 years old, but you'd never know it. In fact he could be any age. He stands about five feet, nine inches tall. He's about average build but very compact, and at this point in his life, as thin as a sailor who's just come through boot camp. With pale skin and dark hair, in which there is just a hint of gray, he is the kind of man who—while not classically handsome—would nonetheless immediately cause one to turn and take notice of him. He exudes a quiet magnetism, like a man who has something important to do the very next minute, every minute actually. His impeccable clothes suggest a classic sense of style—Eastern establishment rather than Texas developer—wing-tipped shoes, conservative suits and ties. The only odd thing is the perpetual unlighted cigar, always there in his hand or mouth. It's cut down with a knife now, as if its size is disappearing as he "smokes" it. The cigar is a prop left over from earlier days, important to Fred's identity; common gestures include waving it through the air to punctuate remarks in his conversation or holding it between two fingers as he slams his fist down on a table to emphasize a point.

I asked Fred how he happened to end up in Houston in the construction business. I knew only that he is of Lebanese descent and had once owned a carpet-cleaning business in Los Angeles.

"And a delicatessen," he adds. "I'm originally from Des Moines, Iowa. During the Second World War, I was in the Pacific and so I went to L.A. first after the service. I went to UCLA and then to Drake University, although I never finished high school."

"I picked Houston," he continues, "because I didn't know anybody here. Before law school classes started I made a living bartending. I had built one apartment complex, sort of an investment for my parents. I was so far in debt on the first building, I continued to build more. I finished law school, passed the bar and got so tied up in apartments that it was impossible for me to ever practice law."

I asked if he came from a big family.

"I have five brothers, let's see . . ." He stops to count, "One, two, three, yes, five brothers, two are dead. Three are still alive. They live here in Houston. My mother and father also came here to live. They've both passed away."

"And you brought a lot of family over from Lebanon," I probed.

He pooh-poohs the question. "I brought some family over from Lebanon and a lot of non-family over too. I didn't really bring them over as such. I helped some of them come over."

"And didn't you help them get started?"

"Quite a few of them," he answers absently.

Although Fred is noncommittal about his role in supporting family and friends, on a previous trip I had been escorted by a young Lebanese woman who had just arrived in the United States and was working in Fred's office until she could go to business school. She described a number of instances in which Fred Rizk had helped people become established in this country.

Before I can ask any more questions, Fred says, "I thought we were going to talk about Pritikin. Why do you want to know about me?" I explained to him that people will also want to know about him personally. He grunts, as if the thought makes no sense to him.

We complete another couple of laps around the track. It's beginning to get dark and Fred decides it's time to quit. We dart back into the building and head for the locker room lobby, where we run into one of Fred's friends. He and Fred exchange a few words. The friend is overweight and Fred mentions the Pritikin diet. "You should give it a try, Coz," he says. The friend nods, but each of us knows the advice is worthless. We separate and I shower, change and dry my hair. Meeting again at the reception desk, Fred and I walk out into a beautiful Texas night, climb into the steel-gray Mercedes coupe and head for home and dinner.

Sylvia Rizk is a very rare person. A dark-haired, dark-eyed beauty, in her late thirties, she incongruously seems to possess the wisdom of the ages. She has been married to Fred for six years—met him "at work." Today, she directs the management side of Fred's business. Simply put, he builds the apartments, she keeps them full and maintained. It's a hectic job in a hectic industry, but to look at her sitting with her infant son in her arms, you would think she has done nothing else with her life but raise children. It's no secret to anyone who knows and loves Fred that he is a whirling dervish of activity. He drives his people hard, not only for his own needs but in the service of others. Making arrangements for my recent trip to Houston, for example, he insisted I stay at his home and he sent one of his junior secretaries to fetch me from the airport, rent me a car and deliver me to the Rizk house.

Carol, my airport escort, filled me in about Fred's car accident and the new baby. When the news was exhausted, we swapped stories about Fred's "craziness." The interesting thing is that when people talk about the pace Fred Rizk keeps, the mood is more often wonderment than criticism. It is no secret to me, however, that my sanity wouldn't last long around this maelstrom of thoughts, feelings, activities and emotions. So I wonder how Sylvia does it. She moves like a calm breeze through the middle of this activity, offering fresh insights, listening to Fred's plans and schemes, straightening conflicting schedules and demands and making practical and well-founded comments. Sometimes her husband listens, sometimes he doesn't. I suspect he listens more often than not, but nobody seems to be keeping score. She calls him Bear or the Middle Eastern Habebe—the Lebanese influence is still heavy in the Rizk household. Most times, he calls her Hon.

On our way home, as we stop at a traffic light, Fred finishes describing the accident that temporarily incapacitated his Mercedes. "I was talking on the car phone," he concludes, "didn't even have time to hang up." Another Mercedes pulls up on our passenger side. Fred eases my window down with the power switch on his console. "How's it coming, Coz?" he shouts across at the man in the adjacent car. (I remember to stop trying to figure out who really is a "Coz.") The man next to us answers with a tirade of explanations about paint and parts and delays, delivered in a slightly foreign accent. "OK, but quick, huh?" Fred shouts back. "I've got to get this car back to Sylvia." The man in the other car turns out to be Fred's mechanic. I think to myself, "Houston's a big city. What are the chances of this happening? Who would look for it to happen?" But Fred Rizk acts like this is a small town and he's the mayor.

Dinner is on the table when we arrive home. Fred and Sylvia and I eat and talk about everything from the Pritikin Program to real estate deals and the state of the economy. The Rizk kitchen is the house's command post. Although there's a phone a few feet away in the den, Fred uses the one on a shelf behind him, level with the height of the dining table. The phone is an extension of Fred's senses, in use constantly. An idea dawns and he picks up the phone. A question arises, he remembers who might have the answer and reaches for the telephone. If he doesn't get the answer the first time, he plugs in another call. Tonight we're discussing the availability of tickets for tomorrow's horse show. He dials, his contact can't be reached, which puts the subject temporarily on hold. The particularly fascinating aspect of Fred's phone manner is that he doesn't hesitate for a moment before applying finger to touchtone dial. He seems not to consider whether this might not be the proper time to call, nor worry that the party might not be in nor be inspired to hear from him. His telephone style is a symptom of an important personality characteristic—in a fundamental sense, Fred Rizk is an impatient man who prefers immediate gratification to prolonged deliberation.

The doorbell rings. Some elegantly dressed friends have come to see new baby, Rex. We sit and talk as Sylvia opens the gifts they've brought. Fred serves food and drink, explains what he's putting in front of them. The guest are Lebanese, so Fred pushes the lentils. We talk about heart disease and diet and Fred suggests his guests investigate the Pritikin diet. They promise to look into it. It's about eleven o'clock when they leave and I decide to call it a day. Fred, however, will probably be awake until one, watching old movie westerns on TV. One evening I came home late only to catch Fred in front of the small black-and white portable on the shelf next to the kitchen telephone. I sat down, and for a while, we both watched James Stewart match wits with John Wayne in *The Man Who Shot Liberty Valance*. Sylvia had long since called it a day. Tired, I also gave up before the movie was over and had to be briefed the next morning. Fred, of course, filled me in. It was probably the fourth or fifth time he'd seen the film.

Sunday afternoon found us back in Sylvia's Mercedes, driving toward the outskirts of Houston, headed for the arena and the horse show. Fred is dressed in a madras plaid shirt over exquisitely tailored cotton slacks, his outfit finished with black cowboy boots. It is another hot summer Texas day. The Mercedes purrs quietly along the amazingly uneven Houston roads, its powerful air conditioning protecting us from the heat outside. As I begin to ask questions, it's obvious that Fred is uneasy—but won't say so—about how much "research" I'll require. This day, he anticipates my successive questions. The answers come in a punctuated rhythm.

"Are you a perfectionist?" I ask.

"I am," he answers precisely.

"Are you hard on people?" I press.

"On myself and other people, particularly myself."

"Where do you think that comes from?"

"Probably wanting to achieve."

"Where did you get that," I pursue, "from your family?"

"Not at all," he says blandly.

"Are you second generation?"

"Yes I am."

"So your parents were immigrants," I conclude. "What did your father do?"

"He was a salesman of imported linens."

"Did your father ever give you any message about succeeding?"

"No," says Fred. "He always thought education was very important—because he didn't have that."

"So where did you get this perfectionist thing from? Do you know?"

"Oh, I think it's a matter of trying to achieve," he responds. "I was never an achiever in school."

"You didn't like school?"

"Hated it."

"How did you get through law school if you hated school?"

"Well, I realized there was only one way I could use a B.S., and I didn't particularly want to waste it. So I went to law school. I felt that I liked law and I thought I could do well in it."

"Did you play any sports in high school?"

"No."

"Nothing really turned you on?"

"No. I didn't finish high school," he reminds me. "I went into the service before I finished, so I missed a couple of years. And when I got out of the service I thought I was too old for college. I worked for four years, then I decided that I needed an education and ought to have one. That's when I started college."

"What did your father think when you didn't finish high school?"

"It didn't make much difference," Fred says and then adds, "I didn't particularly care what people cared or thought at that time."

The roof of the arena that is our destination is beginning to show itself against the low Texas sky. "Were you always so independent?" I asked.

"Very," he answers, "even with five brothers."

"Were you the oldest, youngest?"

"I was the youngest." Then he adds, "I think I'm sort of the black sheep of the family." He stops, rethinks it then and says, "I shouldn't say that, I'm different from the other brothers. Much more . . ."

But the thought is lost. We're at the entrance to the arena. Fred's attention shifts to a group of people who are gathered around the entrance gate—each with specific duties to sell tickets, collect money or provide parking directions. There also seems to be a few hangers-on just enjoying the day. Fred asks if any tickets are being held for us. Two of the young people shuffle through some envelopes. No, there are no tickets. Fred's contact has failed. "How much are they?" he asks, pulling out some loose bills. The young person sells him two tickets and starts to give him the change. "Forget it," Fred says. "Give it to whatever this thing's for."

We drive past the kids, who look a little confused, and find a place to park. It's cool in the open-air arena, out of the sun. The sod interior is moist and some of its coolness is reflected off the cinder blocks and concrete that line the grandstands. I foolishly expect that we'll sit and watch the competition. The horses are jumpers, on a circuit sponsored by Mercedes-Benz and Rolex watches. Fred scans the area. He can't find the people he's looking for. We head toward the hospitality suite, located at one end of the arena. People are lined up along windows, viewing the action. His friends are not here either, but Fred and I move closer to a window just in time to see the horse and rider that are the object of our trip. She does well, with only one jumping fault, but that will put her out of the second-round finals. We agree that her performance was impressive. Fred asks me if I'd like a drink. I decline. This takes all of five minutes, and we are off again in search of his friends, this time down the stairs on the opposite side of the hospitality area.

Here we meet with success—horse, rider and coach, the man we've been looking for—standing together in the staging area. We congratulate the young horsewoman. Fred engages in some shop talk with her coach. I wander away from them, lean on a fence and watch the action. Horses and riders pace back and forth in the warm-up area behind me, waiting their turn. It's hotter down here, the sun shines on our backs, and there's a smell of horseflesh and warm bodies. Fred comes over and watches; we spend another five minutes watching quietly, but in a minute we're off to the grandstands, passing the food concessions as we go. Fred notes that before Pritikin he would have stopped and bought a couple of candy bars; today, we blithely move on. Down front, we sit and are introduced to other owners and riders. Again I start to watch the competition as Fred takes a seat in the row in front of me. The contest becomes exciting as the first round nears completion and the jumping becomes more intense. Turning around in his seat, Fred says, "You really like this stuff, huh?" I laugh, wondering vaguely where we'll be off to next.

Forty minutes later, the jumping over, we leave early to beat the traffic, driving back toward the city through the Texas landscape that stretches flat for miles in all directions. The car holds the road nicely, and Fred seems to be concentrating on the wheel. He hasn't made a phone call yet. I watch the fields go by, here and there populated with billboards proclaiming new housing developments. Fred points to a piece of land on the right of the highway. "This," he says, "is the type of land I used to own. I had twenty pieces of land this good."

From previous experience, I knew of Fred's disgust with missed opportunity, but I ask what happened anyway.

"Lost it," he says. "Had to sell."

The absent way he answers the question makes me wonder how these things come about, so I ask how he pulls out of something like that.

"Worked my butt off," he says and then goes on to describe what might be called the essential Rizk philosophy. "When I have a problem, I don't give up," he explains. "I just work harder. If you continue to fight, you're going to win sooner or later. Never give up; once you give up, once you hesitate, you're gone." He pauses, his right hand is on the wheel, his left elbow on the armrest, in his hand the ever-present cigar. "So I'm back to where I was. Most of my stuff is for other things and other people anyhow. I don't need any more money, I just need stuff to do. You can only buy so much and take a chance on so much. I don't go into a piece of land now unless I'm quite sure I have a partner with me that can weather the storm. What happened last time was most of my partners went broke and I had to carry their share and mine, but I never foreclosed with my partners. I used to always go for the underdog. I still do."

I ask why. "I put myself in that position," he explains. "I was never the top of anything, the top of the class, the top of nothing."

To my suggestion that he is now, Fred responds, "I know, but I'm

still for the underdog.'' The next second, he realizes what we're talking
about. "But this doesn't have anything to do with Pritikin," he says
closing the conversation.

Quickly changing the subject I asked Fred what perpetrated his
decision about bypass surgery.

"I had the angiogram in November," he reflects, "and I woke up
early New Year's morning and the pain in my chest was really bad. It
must have lasted probably thirty minutes, but it seemed like hours. I
was scheduled for bypass surgery in January because my doctor felt that
it was important that I get it done. Denton Cooley was going to do the
surgery."

Unsatisfied with the results of drug treatment, Fred's doctors recommended the bypass they had identified as a possibility at the time of
his angiogram. Their recommendation, however, didn't sit well with
Fred. "I had been thinking about it for some time," he continues. "The
day for the surgery kept getting closer and closer and the pains weren't
any less." The dull tone of his voice seems to convey a continued sense
of puzzlement about the course of events during that time of his life. He
continues, "I literally made up my mind [against surgery] the day
before I actually went out to the Pritikin center. I said, 'We're going to
take that chance and see what happens.'

"I was depressed," he recalls, "and I was angry that this could
happen to me. I was angry because I had never known what was really
going on with the food, with the way I was eating. I was not frightened
of an operation," he insists. "I had a hernia operation about two years
after Pritikin and I went through it as smooth as hell. But I just hated
the idea of somebody touching my goddamn body because of food.
And I knew it was food.

"I was basically mad at myself," he maintains. "I didn't know
any different. But who was I to blame? You can only blame yourself.
And I was scared," he concedes openly. "I was so scared of what
might happen that for a long time when I went to bed at night, I'd just
pray for the urge that woke me up—that bathroom call. When I got up
for that, I knew I'd make it through the night. I had a lot of anxiety,"
he concedes, "months and months and months. I'd go to sleep and I'd
just want to get that wake-up call. Once I got through that wake-up, I
knew I'd make it."

"It was awful," he recalls, an uncharacteristic softness in his
usually deep, gruff voice. "It really was. Also, every night for a long
time, I had my nitroglycerin with me wherever I went, never went
without it for years—at least two years. Even after Pritikin I did that,
for not quite a year, although I felt much better then."

I asked Fred if he took an intellectual inventory before he made his decision not to have bypass surgery.

His answer is simple. "I just figured that I was either going to cure myself or that was going to be it, period. I had made my mind up. I could say that I didn't want my chest screwed up, but that's not the reason. The real reason was that I wouldn't be a man, a real man with bypasses in me." He pauses, I wait, and he repeats the thought again. "As far as I'm concerned, I wouldn't feel like a real man. I didn't want my body screwed with." And then he adds the familiar words, "It would be a loss of control. A loss of control of my own body."

"And you saw the Pritikin Program as a chance to get some control back?" I asked quietly.

"Yes, I did. I felt that there was a real chance of reversal of atherosclerosis. But I felt it would take a minimum of two years. People I was with at the Pritikin center would ask if they'd be all right in twenty-six days. I thought that was silly. You can't screw a body up for fifty years and then try to undo it in twenty-six days.

"Actually in my case, my diet probably became bad when I went in the service and started eating the junk food when I was on liberty. And then the pace and the way I ate . . . I really screwed my life up in the last thirty-five years."

So Fred Rizk declined to join the ranks of Henry Kissinger, Danny Kaye, Walter Matthau and the some one million other Americans who have elected to have bypass surgery. The number of surgeries performed seems to suggest that bypass surgery is a simple operation. In fact, it takes six to ten weeks to recuperate from the immediate physical effects of the surgery and fully six months to a year to completely recover. A large percentage of bypass patients do not return to their previous employment after surgery, and a great many patients experience severe mental stress and depression for months after the procedure. In *Bypass—A Doctor's Recovery From Open Heart Surgery*, Connecticut psychologist Joseph Wayberg tells of his own inability to deal with the emotional effects of bypass surgery and of his experiences forming consciousness-raising groups for fellow patients and their wives. People unfamiliar with someone who has experienced bypass surgery and its effects might find it easy to dismiss Fred's apprehension as inconsequential. The truth is that many post-bypass patients, when questioned, have admitted ambivalence about having elected to have the surgery. With this in mind, I asked Fred how he came to discover the Pritikin Program.

"I had a friend in Los Angeles," he explains, "an attorney, who had read where some airline pilots had gone to the Pritikin center to be recertified. He sent me the Pritikin book and I started studying it. It made a lot of sense to me. All I had to do was follow a typical day of what I ate and I could see that I was doing everything wrong. It made a lot of sense that when you eat grease, it's going to clog up your arteries. But," he reveals, "I'd never thought about that before, never heard of it before."

His doctor, he says, was concerned about the severity of Fred's case but noncommittal about the Pritikin Program. "He said they had done a study where they took some patients who were having angina and put them in a hotel for a month, fed them lowfat food, had them on yoga and exercise and they became less and less dependent on nitroglycerin. And their angina decreased. After I heard about the Pritikin Program, I asked my doctor about it. He didn't discourage me, but he felt that mine was a rather critical case. I was having pains at rest that's the worst kind."

Although his doctor was not enthusiastic about recommending the Pritikin Program, Fred—ever straining at the limits—found encouragement from another area. "After I had the angiogram," he reveals, "I decided to talk to Dr. Donald Wukasch. I knew him from business and also socially. I told him about my problem and asked him to read my records. He concurred about the amount of blockage, that I had the three vessels blocked. He said I had a fifty-fifty chance with the Pritikin Program, because a lot depended, not just on modifying the food I ate, but on whether or not I could break through that critical barrier between starting to exercise and the point at which I would build collateral circulation. He felt that if I could get through that period, then I had a chance. His other point was that personality has a lot to do with the success of the program—how well you try and whether or not you can change your life-style. Because to be successful with this, you've got to change your whole way of life, not just the food, but also your temperament. That's the hardest thing for me to do, and I have not done it. I've tempered it some, but not very much."

Dr. Donald Wukasch is currently the medical director of the LivingWell-Houstonian Preventative Medicine Center, which is attached to the health club where Fred works out. At the time of Fred's angiogram and subsequent decision-making, however, Dr. Wukasch was an associate of Dr. Denton Cooley at the Texas Heart Institute, where he was coordinator for clinical service and himself a cardiac surgeon. Although involved in conventional approaches to heart disease, Dr. Wukasch was also interested in the work of Nathan Pritikin. "I very much supported the idea of Fred's attempting the Pritikin Program," says Wukasch. "I thought he could do it and I thought it would be good for him. And it has been. Fred's was a fairly critical case because of the blockage in the left anterior descending artery and the diagonal branch of the circumflex artery. That put that whole left area of Fred's heart at risk. Now, you have to remember that at that time it was not accepted that atherosclerosis could be reversed and so there was the question of whether it was justifiable to withhold surgery. Fred's doctor had recommended the bypass as the most conservative medical approach.'' Wukasch also remembers that Denton Cooley wasn't happy that Fred decided against surgery. Since Fred's experience, however, Dr. Wukasch has personally referred numbers of people to the Pritikin Program. "We have learned," he says, "that everyone doesn't have to have bypass surgery, that many people are better treated with life-style change, but at that time I was literally putting my reputation on the line. I told Fred, 'You're risking your life, but if you drop dead out there, my whole professional career will be on the line.' '' Dr. Wukasch continues to support the Pritikin Program and has remained an informal source of help and guidance to Fred.

When I asked Fred what he meant by his remark of "tempering" his life-style, he answers, "Well, that means get to a B personality," as if the idea were so obvious that I should be faulted for asking. "At least an A personality," he says. "Right now, I'm a triple A. One time when I saw Gotto [one of the cardiologists he consulted], he reached up and got the A behavior book and gave it to me. He knew what I was like from just talking to me. He said, 'Read this.' So I read it and gave it back to him. It didn't do me any good," he concludes.

"You see," Fred continues, "I didn't quite agree with the type A personality. Although it's a factor, I didn't think it was directly related to blockage and neither did Pritikin. And there's some new evidence coming out now that proves he was right. Your behavior doesn't have as much effect on the heart as people think. But I have always tried to make a conscious effort. I keep trying. And I think I've improved quite a bit. I try," he explains, "not to get as serious when there are mistakes."

"You mean laugh more?" I asked.

"No," he answers. "Just try to walk away from things. I mean, a mistake is not going to be corrected by raising hell about it."

Although Fred Rizk had been considering alternatives for bypass for some time, he decided to tell no one of his decision to skip the surgery and try the Pritikin Program. The day before he was scheduled to check into the hospital for the bypass, Fred—the man to whom the telephone is second nature—asked a friend to call his physician's office to apprise him that "Fred couldn't make the surgery," as if it were simply one additional appointment in a chronically overcrowded schedule. Fred contends he utilized this strategy because he feared risking the possibility that "my doctor might talk me into it." The phone call made, Fred boarded a plane to Los Angeles.

Once at the Pritikin center, he established long-distance telephone arrangements with his office and expresses pride at the fact that he didn't neglect his business affairs "even one day" while he was at the center. Although at the time he made his decision against bypass, Fred was engaged to marry Sylvia, he did not inform her in advance of his plans. He admits, however, that she would have been supportive of his decision. When I suggested that Sylvia didn't appear to be the kind of person to abandon him because of his illness, he answered simply, "She wouldn't have; it was me."

Sylvia and Rubie, Fred's cook at that time, eventually spent the last week with him at the Santa Monica Pritikin Center. Nine months after Fred left the center, he and Sylvia were married. Of the wedding, he says, "I should have done it ten years ago. We'd have had two or three kids by now."

If one can credit the opinion of his wife, Fred and Sylvia Rizk had what could be called a circuitous courtship—an on-again, off-again romance undoubtedly complicated by their hectic business schedules and commitments. Although Fred is quick to attribute his concern about marrying Sylvia to his problems with heart disease, she, in her unself-conscious way, has another explanation. While Fred may rationalize that he didn't want to tie her down to a sick man who might die suddenly, Sylvia remembers things differently. "Fred loved being engaged," she says, rolling her large brown eyes and laughing. "He just loved it. After a lot of back and forth, I had finally decided I wanted to marry him. So we got engaged. And he liked that a lot." Sylvia says she doesn't recall being concerned about the liabilities of Fred's health. She speaks about his visit to the Pritikin center and his commitment to the program as if it's simply part of the man who is Fred Rizk. And Fred rightfully credits her with his impressive rate of adherence to the program. "There's one thing that's very important to say," he reminds me, "the support of the person who's closest to you. I couldn't have done it without her." Sylvia is nonchalant about her acceptance of the diet. "You know," she says, "sometimes when we're traveling and I've had a few rich meals, I have to go back to eating Pritikin, because I feel so heavy and uncomfortable." There are no soapboxes in the Rizk household, no elaborate routines to assure adherence, just simple acceptance that this is the way it is.

In the car on our way back to the city, we have slipped back into personal territory again, and as with all questions that he feels touch on private areas, Fred chisels away at his answers.

I ask what he thought about Sylvia during the time he was making his decision between Pritikin and bypass surgery.

"I didn't think it was fair to her to marry her," he answers forthrightly. "I didn't know what the hell was going to happen to me. I didn't know if I was going to make it or not."

"What did she think?" I asked.

"I think she felt I could," he says. "I mean, she didn't care." That's not what he means and rephrases his answer. "I mean she cared but she was willing to take the chance."

I ask about the reactions of other people in his life when he came back from the Pritikin center.

"Many, many people said they thought I wouldn't make it," he remembers. "That I should have had the bypass. Many of them, however, ended up eating their words. Later I talked about it with them when they were better informed, when they were starting to believe in it a little bit. Even after the second angiogram, they didn't believe that there was any possibility of regression. I wasn't irritated by these people a bit, not a bit," he finishes quickly. "I didn't give a damn what they thought. Still don't."

The car purrs along quietly over the bumpy highway. We're both silent. As we approach the suburbs of the city, Fred breaks the silence. He looks at me and says, as if my probing hasn't been as bad as he thought it might be, "You know, hon, you're all right."

II

"I don't know if I could ever be satisfied with anything I've done."

Back in town, Fred and I decided to stop in a coffee shop for something cold to drink. By then, it was a late Sunday afternoon and people were arriving for dinner. The hostess had a problem understanding that we just wanted to sit and talk. Finally she showed us to an out-of-the-way booth. A waitress brought diet sodas with lots of ice. I realized that if I were ever to catch Fred in a reflective moment, this might be it. At first his thoughts were delivered in his usual curt fashion, but gradually he allowed himself to explore his opinions and recollections further.

Easing into the conversation, I began with the "Pritikin" questions. I wanted to know if he had foreseen what it would be like before he went to the Pritikin center and what he did when he got there.

"No, I didn't," he answers easily, "but once I was there, I was a very serious, serious patient. I've always taken any medical advice very seriously. I was extremely conscientious while I was there because I was very worried. When I was at the center," he continues, "I was friendly with a bunch of people, but I did my own workouts. I did my own thing."

The sodas arrive, and the waitress makes a great deal of effort delivering napkins and straws. Taking a sip of his drink, Fred points the habitual cigar directly at me to emphasize what he's about to say. "I didn't cheat while I was at the center and I didn't cheat for two years, and I mean, I didn't cheat." He enunciates these words very clearly, pausing to give each one equal emphasis. "You can ask her," he continues, "she'll tell you. I was on the Regression Diet for two years—no meat. I'm talking about not one piece of candy." He leans back against the booth. "Unbelievable—two years."

Continuing his testimony, he says, "Gotto was talking to Wukasch one day, and he said, 'I've only one patient that could stay on the Pritikin diet.' Gotto wouldn't tell him who the patient was. But Wukasch asked if it was Fred Rizk, and Gotto said, 'Yes.' "

I wondered if Fred felt sorry for himself while he was at the center.

"No," he answered quickly, "not a bit. I didn't miss a lecture. I had friends in California that I'd known for seems like fifty years. I didn't see any of them. I told them if they wanted to come see me at the center that was fine. But I wouldn't miss a day. I didn't go to anybody's house until, I think, the last day or two. I didn't ever go out to eat. I never took the chance. I wanted to make sure that everything I ate was perfect. And while I was at the center, I got off all my medications.

"I had been working out on the Pritikin Program with the book," he remembers. "Walking mostly. I couldn't jog yet. I was walking ten miles twice a week, minimum. And I walked about five or six miles every day. I did much more than what Pritikin asked for in the book. I kept it up and I kept getting better every day. Then I started jogging gradually. At the center I would walk three minutes, jog one minute. I never did get to a steady jog while I was there.

"Jogging was something I wanted to do," he explains, "because I knew that my heart rate would be better that way. And the food didn't bother me a bit. I could have cared less. I used to take people's dinner that they couldn't eat. I was hungry all the time, even towards the end."

Working with the Pritikin book, Fred had dropped his cholesterol almost 100 points, from the high 200s down to 172. "The only thing I was wrong on," he reflects, "was the amount of chicken we could eat, and I thought I could eat commercial granola." When I remind him that commercial granola is loaded with sugar, he responds longingly, "God, I love it, though. But I got off of that. Now I'll eat a little bit with my regular cereal."

The dietary program mastered, Fred turned his attention to exercise. "After I got out of the center, I got to where I was jogging six miles four days a week," he explains, "and two days a week I would jog four miles. They were usually ten-minute miles. And along with that I would also walk some. I don't know how many miles. I used [Kenneth] Cooper's book. His theory is that you only need thirty points to condition your heart. My minimum was ninety points a week, and I would go as high as 125, 130 points. That's why my weight went all the way down to 140. I was eating and eating and eating and couldn't gain weight. I only started to gain a little weight after I went on the Maintenance Diet."

Again, he leans back against the booth, gathering momentum for his next thought. It comes rapidly, punctuated with sweeps of the unlit cigar. "I know now that if I'd known about Pritikin twenty years earlier, there's no way in hell I would let myself get in that shape." The look in his eye and the determination in his voice leaves no doubt that he means it. "At forty-five years old," he continues, "until I ruptured a disk in my back, I was one hell of a judo player, and I mean a hell of one. I have gotten hurt, but it was a great workout for me. It was the greatest workout in the world, just the greatest. That's the only workout I really and truly liked, and I can't do that now because of my back. I don't have any pleasure in walking or bicycling or swimming," he reveals. "It's a routine, part of my life, like brushing my teeth."

He stops just a moment and then says conclusively, his statement reminiscent of Jack Rutta's bravado, "I was damn good for my age, and any place I went in the world nothing scared me and nobody scared me."

When I asked Fred if he still feels that way, the answer is quick. "No," he says, "I don't have that now. In other words, I'll get into a physical battle at sixty years old with almost anyone, but I know I haven't got it, you see. It's a matter of pride, not just ability. More than anything, it's hard for me to back down.

"If had to fight and it was to the death," he continues, "I was prepared to do it. That was my way, I always felt that way. I should have been born a couple hundred years ago," he says pensively. "I would have made a hell of a revolutionary." He stops, pours what's left of the diet soda over the remaining ice in the plastic glass. "I didn't hesitate back then but I would hesitate now, I'm afraid, and hesitation is what kills you." Then he adds still another poignant thought. "I'm a determined enough individual, although I feel a little differently, now that I have a child."

"Are you getting more mellow as you get older?" I asked him.

For some reason, the question strikes a chord and he says with a grin, "If you shut that thing off, I'll tell you." The flag is up—we're moving into non-Pritikin territory again. I withdraw my question and ask him instead if he was totally prepared to implement the diet and exercise program full-time after he left the center.

"I was," he responds grimly. "I did. I did for two solid years and I can say today that in six-and-a-half years I have not had a meal, other than desserts, that is incorrect. I can say that, and I can say that the rest of my life will be the same way. Because I could care less about food." I grin, and from my previous experiences with Fred, acknowledge the strength of his resolution. He concludes his testimony with a committed flourish, "No, you don't have to worry about me; I'll be straight."

"So you don't have to continually commit yourself to the diet?" I pressed. "No," he answers, "I just assume I'm on it. I never think about it. I have accepted it as a way of life and I have no problem with it. In fact once in a while we'll have people to dinner and we will get food other than Pritikin. If I had my way and if it were up to me, when I entertain, all my food would be Pritikin. Nothing else. When I went to the Pritikin center, I made my commitment then."

Two years, almost to the day, after he left the Pritikin Longevity Center in Santa Monica, Fred Rizk had a second angiogram. As he describes it, he had been on the diet faithfully for two solid years and his doctors had accepted his commitment to the Pritikin Program—and his impressive results. But Fred wanted proof that he had chosen the right course. "I wanted to know," he says. "I was going crazy.

"I felt good," he explains. "My treadmills were good. I was on a treadmill at the doctor's office for thirty-two minutes. He told me, 'You don't need to do this; your heart is fine.' But," Fred confides, "he was kind of curious, too. After it was over, he came in the room, and he said to me, 'Well, it's never been done before, but the ninety's down to forty. There is some regression.' He was surprised, but he could believe it, determined as I was. I really was loyal to the diet and still am. I still almost go crazy if something is wrong with my food." As illustrated by his first angiogram, Fred had ninety percent closure of one of the secondary branches of his left coronary artery. He is referring here to the fact that after two years on the Pritikin Program, the blockage had been reduced to less than half of what it was. Additionally the sixty percent blockage in the main branch of the left artery was also reduced, almost by half.

Among Pritikin circles, it was generally considered that Fred's double angiograms were testimony to the effect of the Pritikin program. In the face of continued criticism from the medical establishment for data verifying his claims, Nathan Pritikin had hoped that the results of the Rizk angiograms might be developed as a scientific case study, and, in fact, a paper was written on Fred's experience. However, the fact that the two angiograms were not completed under identical circumstances and at the same facility negated them as scientifically verifiable evidence. Retaining his interest in the Pritikin Program, Dr. Wukasch co-authored the case study with Dr. Donald Rochelle of the Texas Heart Institute (Fred's original cardiologist), who had also seen Fred as a patient; Nathan Pritikin; and Dr. James Bernard of UCLA and the Pritikin Research Foundation. Regardless of the outcome of the paper, the second angiogram reinforced Fred's belief in the program.

I ask him if after the second angiogram, he went out and celebrated. But celebrations aren't Fred's thing. "I'm not too much on celebrations," he says. "Every day's a celebration, see. Every day I'm here is a celebration. But I felt great, great. I had no pain. The pain became less and less and less after I left Pritikin. Only once in a while would it come back but never when I was at rest. Only when I was doing too much physically or when I was angry."

I wondered what kind of anger he's referring to.

He cuts me off sharply. "In this business—you've never been in the construction business or you'd realize how often you can get angry. It's just one of those types of businesses. Can you imagine having 700 to 1,000 apartment units all going at one time?" He changes the subject. "The pain back then was only when I was stressed or extra tired. And I never have slept well—five or six hours a night. I've been trying to take naps and usually I'll get maybe three a week in. When I first came back from the center, I got at least twenty minutes of rest a day. I would try to meditate twenty minutes, lying down every afternoon."

The coffee shop is starting to fill up and the noise is making it difficult to talk. We leave our empty glasses, pay the check, and slide back into the car, headed for Sylvia's parents' home. Five minutes into our ten-minute ride, Fred picks up the phone and starts pressing buttons. "Hi," he says to someone on the other end of the line. "How do you feel?" He waits patiently. "Now don't get upset," he says. "We'll help you with it. What you've got to do is get out there during the day and sell.'' The conversation ends after a few more words of fatherly advice.

Fred puts the phone back in its cradle and explains. ''That was a friend of ours. Sylvia told me she's been having trouble with her business. We're going to help her get back on her feet. She can do it, she just needs a little help.'' He says all of this very matter-of-factly, as though such activities are an accepted part of his life and as if he doesn't have enough to do. We drive a few minutes in silence and he remembers something he wants to tell me.

''Just about a month ago, I danced at high altitude,'' he recalls. ''I love Latin music, and I danced for almost four straight hours in Mexico City. Although I'm in pretty damn good shape, I didn't think, first of all, that I could dance that long. I thought it was three hours and they said four—let's make it three because the Mexicans exaggerated.'' He says this offhandedly; I chuckle. ''Three good, solid hours and then I went home, I didn't know whether I'd make it or not. I didn't feel bad, but your breathing, it's just so hard to breathe up there, and I was tired.'' I ventured that, given what he'd described, I'd be tired.

''No,'' he stops me. ''I do push myself more than most people do. It's my character. If you were to say to me, 'Gee, you have a nice townhouse, or gee, you built a good building,' I would thank you and then I would say, 'It would be fantastic if I'd done this, this, this and this.

''I guess it's that . . .'' He thinks a minute and then says surprisingly, ''I don't know if I could ever be satisfied with anything that I've done. Never. You see, I'm not interested in material things. Those aren't important to me. I don't run around with status things like airplanes and boats, condominiums here, there and all over. I don't need all of that, never really cared for it.''

''What is important?'' I asked him.

The question doesn't throw him, but he's not going to risk formulating an answer before thinking about it. ''That's a tough question,'' he admits.

''Something's got to be important,'' I countered.

Another long moment of reflection stretches between us. I sense that he wants to answer the question but not superficially. ''Tough question,'' he says again. ''What's important?'' he muses to himself. ''Probably what you do with your life.'' He stops again, offers to clarify the thought. ''What you do with your life for others . . . I shouldn't say for other people . . . What you do with your life that you can be proud of.''

There is another long pause. Fred clenches his cigar tightly and looks off into the distance. "I would say . . . what you live for . . . what you can do with your life for the people around you. But then," he adds, "that's sort of narrow. I'd have to get back to you on that. It's a tough one to answer."

Taking one more stab, I asked, "But that's something that does motivate you?"

"That's basically all that does," he answers. "If you leave a good name and you've been successful without screwing somebody, then you've done well. Not very many people are successful and can say that they haven't hurt somebody out there."

I sense in Fred, as in Jack Rutta, a genuine desire to value and respect people. "You like people, don't you?" I asked him.

"Very much."

"You also value people?"

"Yeah I do, very much. But we're going to go into a subject matter that has nothing to do with Pritikin."

So switching gears once again, I ask Fred why he wants to get his cholesterol below his stated goal of 160. Now in familiar territory, he answers unhurriedly, "Because I think I'm not in as good as shape as I was after the first two years." When I look at him askance, knowing Fred's fanaticism about his health, he says, "My treadmill shows everything's good . . . it may just be that I've had some sinus problems the last six, seven months. At one time there was an infection; they got it out and then I started swimming again. And it came right back."

When I suggested that he might be allergic to chlorine, he brightens. "I might be," he says, "and that might be causing my sinus infection. But I'm going to tackle that swimming one way or the other. Because it's the best overall exercise there is." He sneaks a glance my way and confides sheepishly, "And I thought maybe if my back got better, if everything got better with me, I could do the Ironman thing at sixty-some years old." He laughs heartily. It's fun to see Fred smile.

"I'd love to do it," he grins, "and if I had a good back, I'd do it. I can't run . . . but I could walk it. See, I could walk twenty-six miles now, if I had to, with no trouble." He thinks about the idea a minute longer, and likes it. "It'd be something like hell." I like the idea and agree with him.

We're silent for a minute. "Do you think of yourself now as a heart patient," I asked him, "as somebody with heart disease?"

He rolls the question around for a moment to see how it feels. "I don't feel that . . ." he ruminates and then adds firmly, "no, I really don't." He decides to explain. "Let's say that I knew it, but I didn't accept it. I mean I was worried, but it was hard for me to believe that I could have that problem. I'm finding myself now accepting it, but I still have problems with it. Not that I'm ashamed of it, but just that I don't think in those terms. What brought it home was the last time I went to the Pritikin center. They reduced my workout heart rate because of heart disease. That's when it really started to dawn on me that I really do have a heart problem.

"It affects you unconsciously," he continues, "for quite a while. For example, I didn't exert myself quite as much as I used to—when I first started exercising. I tried to watch my temper more. I really did work at it. But then when you get your confidence up, you start going back to your old habits, which I did. Yes," he says, "I still work as many hours now as before the heart problems. Probably the last eight months is the hardest I've ever worked in my life.

"I don't really want to work that hard," he justifies. "It's just that I need to do it right now. But I think I can cut down within the next thirty days." Then he thinks of something else, and I'm immediately struck by his insight. "Unfortunately, you see, the doctors never tell you how to run your business. They tell you it's not good for you, but they can't tell you what to do about it. In other words, sometimes you get on a roll and you just can't get out of it. You can't just take people who've worked for you for twenty years and say, 'Guys, I'm supposed to slow up. Now you guys find something else to do.' You've got an obligation to the people you work with."

Fred appears to be saying that to be successful with the requirements of the Pritikin life-style modifications he not only has to modify what he eats, but also his expectations. "You should modify your behavior," he says. "That's been the single most difficult thing for me to do. If you can modify your behavior, you've really beat it. Forget the eating; eating is the easiest part. I'm a triple A. If I could just go to a Type A personality, I would have achieved something. I sometimes have as many as 300 calls a day, and I refuse not to return a call." Another notion comes to mind. "You know these gravity hangers that hang you upside down? I tried that for about thirty days. You realize I used to use the phone during the seven to ten minutes I was hanging upside down? You sound different, hanging there, but I wouldn't waste that much time."

"So if I could knock off a couple of As . . . ." he suggests to both of us. Smiling, he concludes, "I would enjoy it. I think it would be much better for me. And I try. I try. Then I just slide back. I try not to get upset over something—mistakes. Probably the best way to accept them is to remember that this happens every day, with everybody in the world. I've got the most efficient group in the world, when you compare me with the government—maybe not if you compare me with other companies.''

I asked what he thinks of work. ''Some work is fun,'' he answers, and then goes on to describe the satisfaction he's received from his type of work. ''Well, let's say I've gotten to the point now where I'm sort of burned out on building. I'm going to cut that down to a minimum. I used to love building. I used to love to watch something grow. Most of my buildings I designed myself. I don't do that anymore and it's no fun if you don't design them—they're not yours. It's not something you created yourself. I still like developing land, seeing what I can do with it. When I developed the Three Fountains area, I had 140 acres. I designed it so one area would be townhouses and one apartments; so there'd be a shopping center and offices. There was absolutely nothing out there. People thought I was nuts, but the development happened just like that. So that's fun; I still like to do that.

''What I'll do now will be fun work; I'll be able to go out of town and not come back the same day. And it'll be sort of a fun thing—looking at land, deciding what I can do with it, deciding what . . .'' His thought is cut off as we arrive at Sylvia's parents. Spotting a small red import belonging to Sylvia's sister, Fred again launches into his resolution to return his wife's car to her. This seems to be more of a problem for him than Sylvia, who doesn't appear to be complaining about not having her automobile. Our visit with Fred's in-laws lasts a quick thirty minutes. Sylvia's mother and father are retired. Both easy-going people, they seem to have adjusted long ago to Fred's energy level. As I sit and drink a glass of water, Sylvia's father shows me the scars from his bypass surgery. ''My legs still hurt,'' he tells me. ''They ache sometimes.''

Somehow, during our multi-sided conversation, Fred managed to locate whole wheat bread and bananas and has made himself a sandwich. Sylvia eventually joined us at the table and rolled her eyes as I pointed to her husband standing with the kitchen phone in his ear, the sandwich in his free hand. He has made at least three calls in less than fifteen minutes. That he can even remember whom he has to call intrigues me. ''You know,'' Sylvia tells me, responding to my observations, ''sometimes I just turn off the phone in my car. It gets him so mad. He yells, 'I was trying to get you. Why didn't you answer?' But sometimes,'' she laughs good-naturedly, in her soft Southern drawl, ''I just can't stand it.''

The next day is Monday and a business day, packed, as Fred's days usually are, with nonstop appointments. The schedule calls for him to pick me up on his way home at a hotel where I'm visiting friends. By the time he arrives at the hotel, it's after seven o'clock. I'm ready to go home, take off my shoes and sit down to some dinner. Fred has other plans.

"Hi, hon," he shouts from the car. "Sorry I'm late," he apologizes, swinging up the drive. "How do you feel?" (My appearance must have betrayed me.) I protest that I'm fine. "Good," he says, " 'cause we're going to a restaurant opening."

"Oh God," I groan in the back of my mind, but my picture of the type of restaurant opening Fred Rizk might attend is quickly dispelled. No fancy cuisine this. With Fred recapping his day, explaining to me the various crises he has faced and solved, the big gray car starts through the old streets of the area that was the original downtown Houston. As in many other American cities, this part of town had once been abandoned as its residents flocked to the suburbs. Now, however, it seems to be experiencing a revival, with young artists and trendy groups moving in, looking for lower-cost housing and some sense of inner city sophistication. The streets are narrow and the housing varied, some of the larger houses obviously having been divided into multiple apartments. Fred points out the occasional building he has developed here and there.

Lawns are lush and green and the streets are crowned with a canopy of heavily leafed trees planted years ago to offer shade and still doing their job. The curbs are lined with all manner of cars and Fred worries that the new restaurant will suffer because of lack of adequate parking. "No parking," he says. "That's a problem. I told her that, but she insisted they wanted to do it here." We turn down a small side street off the main artery on which we've been driving, and pull up past a small building that was obviously once a residential cottage. A patio of roughly stained wood juts from the house out to the street on one side of the front door. Next to it, a festive balloon archway welcomes guests. It is altogether a comfortable, homey scene. We drive past the house and Fred pulls into an empty lot where he parks the Mercedes. We walk quickly through the soft Texas dusk to join the crowd already hard at work celebrating the restaurant's opening. The small dining room will specialize in Continental food and will sell wine and food for takeout.

Today's opening, however, offers huge heaping platters of Middle Eastern specialties and jugs of wine. Dressed in a fawn-colored suit, wing-tipped shoes and white shirt, his tie loosened around his unbuttoned collar, Fred moves easily through the crowd with me behind. Everyone knows him. Everybody has a word of greeting to offer. The hands are shaken, the "Coz's" fly back and forth in a hopeless jangle of real and imagined relatives. As well-known as he is to this crowd, and as sought after for a greeting or advice, Fred's movements are somewhat self-conscious, as if he's not totally comfortable being the center of attention. Many of the guests are European or Middle Eastern. As Fred mingles, I munch on a plateful of the delicious food and sip a glass of wine. The place is jammed and Fred finally locates a couple of seats out on the patio. Here I meet Fred's two brothers. One is a gray-haired pediatrician. Dressed in a bow tie and blue-and-white seersucker sport coat, he looks like he just arrived from a small town in New England. Fred and he briefly discuss the new Rizk baby. It's an obsessive topic between the two of them, Fred's intensity predisposing him to anticipate problems with the tiny child before they appear. The second brother is darker complected and looks more European. Dressed in a dark brown suit, he sits among members of the family group with a cane at his knees—holding court.

Fred insists I meet everyone and sample the food, which he refuses to taste. The restaurant's owner, however, has noticed him. She sits him down and tells him to wait for his individually prepared meal. Everybody knows Fred is on a special diet and all make allowances. Despite this, they converse with him on the various nuances of the food on display, knowing that Fred won't sample it.

The crowd continues to grow. Fred is served his special meal and the heavy Texas air begins to lighten as the sun goes down. A few more guests come over to pay their respects, a few more greetings are exchanged, and Fred decides to leave. As we walked back to the car, Fred confided casually, "I had some of my crew come down here and help her out with the building framing and all." Walking a few steps farther, he adds intensely, "God, I hope they make it . . . but the parking . . ."

Back in the car, headed home, Fred calls Sylvia to tell her that we're on the way. We talk leisurely about the business trip he's planning for the next few days. I figure it's now or never for the last few questions.

"What's the worst part about being on the Pritikin diet?" I asked him quickly.

He answers immediately, "Sweets. Maybe once a week I cheat on a candy bar, but where I really go crazy is on yogurt. I'll drive all over town to seek out a place for frozen yogurt. I get a pretty good urge sometimes. It's unbelievable how much I can eat."

Unlike many Pritikin followers, Fred's problem is that his cheating bothers him. "I'm guilty as hell," he says, "just as guilty as you can be.'' I suggested to him that perhaps he should just enjoy it when he slips. ''I wish I could,'' he answers. ''But I can't.''

So even after six years of intermittent falls from the Pritikin wagon, Fred hasn't found a way to adjust to his weakness for sweets. His commitment to the program, however, is complete. Some time ago, he purchased 3,000 copies of one of the Pritikin books to give to friends. I asked how many people he thinks might have taken advantage of the books.

He thinks for a minute, then says, ''Less than five percent.'' Then he admits, ''If I didn't get the scare I did, I don't know whether I could have stuck with it. The scare is almost essential.'' In that light, I asked Fred if he ever feared for his life, feared that he might have a major heart attack and die.

''No, not until after they took the initial angiogram,'' he answers. ''Then I did. Between then and the time I went to Pritikin, yes, I had a great fear of that. My biggest concern was whether I had done what I needed to do for that day. You know—in case I didn't make it to the next day. You try to tie everything up, tie everything down that day. You feel real uncertain, you don't look ahead with any certainty at all.'' He stops and adds, ''You really can't.

''Even today,'' he continues, ''I unconsciously think this way. Unconsciously I'll say, 'There's a few changes in my will I want to make in case something happens.' You never really get it out of your system.''

''The fact that you might . . .'' I suggested.

But he doesn't let me finish. He nods his head. ''Never, really; in fact sometimes even now, once in a while it bothers me if I don't throw a nitroglycerin in my ditty bag when I travel, even though I haven't used them in years. It's like a Linus blanket.

''I've never had a heart attack,'' he goes on. ''But you know how you get funny feelings sometimes—like indigestion can make you feel like it? You can do exercises that hurt your chest and get almost the same feeling. Your neck can hurt in a way and you just wonder, is this the time? Right now I want to take another angiogram, I want to take one so bad I can just hardly wait for it. I want to see, I want to know.

''And if it's not what I want it to be, there's no doubt I would just go on the most determined, determined, determined regression diet that anybody's ever seen. There wouldn't be a human being in the world that would be on a diet like I would. Nobody, not Pritikin, no one. If I had an inkling of fear that it had changed, that the blockage had increased since I took the last one . . . and it would be three hours a day of exercise. I'd either make it again, or I'd break it.''

It's difficult to escape the contradictions of Fred Rizk's personality. He is a person who likes what he's doing but knows the stress it generates can adversely affect his health. An individual who wants to change, but fears he never will. Who wants to drop out of the Type A syndrome, but faces the diet and exercise program that has helped him with the same stressful determination he applies to his work. Sophisticated in his life-style, but engagingly simplistic in his approach to life, he's a caring person, but one quick to anger. A man who is uncompromisingly hard on himself, who will beat himself over the head for a mistake but is generous and can't do enough for other people. Most of all, he is a man impatient for results who has committed himself to a Spartan dietary routine, the effects of which include positive verification in his own mind that the sacrifice is worth it.

"What do you think will happen," I asked, "if you take another angiogram?"

"Don't know," he answers.

"What's your best guess?"

"That it's about the same, the blockage. You see, I don't feel good about myself because I let that cholesterol jump up above 160. I feel bad that I didn't keep it down."

"But you don't feel bad physically?" I asked, aware of Fred's sensitivity to slight nuances in his health.

"No, I feel bad that I didn't keep it down."

"Maybe," I suggested, "you're beating yourself over the head with it."

"I might be," he thinks, "I might be. You know, I've accepted it so strongly . . . that any cheating . . . I feel really guilty. Although it would be nice to get rid of that," he admits, "I can't. I really can't. I don't have that mentality, or that character." (Although the Pritikin cholesterol formula has been specified as 100 plus your age, Dr. Wukasch reminded me that the National Heart Institute and the American Health Foundation both recommend 185 as the magic cholesterol number. Above 185, the risk of developing coronary disease begins to rise.)

I ask Fred if he is someone who enjoys working toward something or if it's the goal that's the most important.

"I think it's the goal," he answers. "It's got to be the goal. That's what that 160 is.

"Now, I can't say I enjoy the Pritikin diet," he continues. "I don't like it at all, but I don't criticize it because I've accepted it. When I was in Africa, I ate the same food for thirty days; the lunch and dinner were the same, the breakfasts were the same and my snacks were the same—cereal and bananas, cereal and bananas. Dinner was rice and vegetables on top, every night, and vinegar and lemon or that Tillie Lewis dressing. That didn't bother me at all. It was just accepted that I had to eat that. I'd take a bite of some animal just to see what it tasted like. It tasted damn good," he admits, "because it didn't have the fat that we have in this country."

He pauses, "I don't know. I'm more of a workaholic than anything else. The means to an end has become an end in itself with me. I don't believe I could ever fully retire," he says. "I think that the work has become an end in itself. I think that I get my satisfaction from that, even though I may say I want to cut down. And I probably will cut down, but I'll substitute something else—probably working out. I'd like to work out about three hours a day.

"And I love traveling, as long as I'm not hopping from one place to another. It is a good substitute; traveling is a good substitute for work. I'm not hunting as often now; I haven't gone in the last year. I used to go for about thirty days. No phones and I got by fine; but you get me anywhere in the states and I couldn't do it. Or anywhere in the world—if I weren't hunting—I couldn't do without a phone."

I ask Fred about his favorite place in the world. If he could spend an unlimited amount of time anywhere, where that might be? He digests my question and replies thoughtfully, "I've been all over the world but as of now I'd say the Greek Islands. It's relaxing; the people are good; it's clean; it's fun to hang around. We've been to Santoríni, Mykonos, Rhodes, although I'll spend more time on the larger islands next time. I think there's more to do there.

"We hike every day. We were going about ten miles every other day, up in the mountains. I'm not a fisherman. You've got to have a lot of patience for fishing. If I'm traveling at fifty miles an hour and I catch a fish every five minutes, I can enjoy it. I'm not a golfer or a fisherman. You've got to give me some action. I'd like to go back to the islands of the Pacific and we'll probably do that next. Also bird hunting in Scotland."

Fred Rizk sits comfortably in the leather seat of the quiet car. The Houston skyline streams by on either side of us, light ricocheting off the windows of the skyscrapers that have made Houston famous. The mood has become somehow serious.

"And then again," Fred says to me, at once crushing the gravity of his previous remarks, "I've yet to go to my first whorehouse." We both laugh. "But," he concludes with conviction, "I'm going to do it before I die."

A Matter of Style

There are two main sitting rooms on the first floor of the Rizk town-house in Houston. One is a beautiful formal living room, finished mostly in European antiques. Light colors and soft materials give the room a feminine feel. A large formal portrait of Sylvia Rizk, dressed in a long gown and flanked by her two Afghan hounds, "The Grey One" and "The White One" as Fred calls them, hangs over the fireplace. The other downstairs public room is a two-story, wood-paneled den, its walls hung with the Rizks' safari trophies. Dominating this room, populated with the heads of gazelles and antelopes and an entire stuffed lion, is a portrait of Fred in safari gear. At once soft and threatening, it captured his intense masculinity and his warm humanity, his impatience and his caring.

The motif in the Rizk corporate office is also of animals. Beautifully carved wooden heads and feet and claws decorate chairs and tables; tapestries of hunting scenes hang on the walls. The virility and vitality of this decor suggest essential elements of Fred Rizk's character. The safari trips continue for the Rizks, more occasionally now, but hunting continues to be a passion.

At work, Fred Rizk continues to maintain a more hectic and goal-oriented pace than Jack Rutta. Fred is more compulsive about his exercise program than Jack. But as Alan Keiser says, "You do what works for you." And it is true that in the long run, a life-style change such as Jack and Fred have undertaken becomes a personal style. The effects are similar, although the effort is different. Rizk and Rutta lead different lives and continue different approaches to the changes in their life necessitated by heart disease. By anyone's standards, however, both are strong, active and involved individuals.

Jack Rutta, for example, has licked the food game. The first time I met him, he was picking over a platterful of party food for something he liked and could eat. He did this, however, in such an effortless manner that I suspected he was after some specially prized tidbit. And just as easily as he sought and located what he wanted to eat, he explained to me why he was doing it—and I had never met him before, nor had I inquired about his behavior that evening.

Bolstered by the success of his bypass surgery, Jack Rutta remains satisfied if his cholesterol stays on the lower end of 200, and he has strategies for adjusting his diet if his cholesterol happens to take a jump into the higher zones. Fred, on the other hand, maintains his commit-ment to keep his level substantially below 200, striving for the Pritikin-recommended target of 100 plus your age. Both men have their cholesterol checked regularly, and Fred's records indicate that he has been generally successful in his quest. His cholesterol continues to stay between 170 and 180.

While both men spend time and energy on exercise, they also approach it in a different way. Jack takes walks during his lunch hour, usually in lieu of eating. Or he rides his stationary bicycle, doing ten miles in twenty-two to twenty-five minutes. When he walks, he figures he does two miles in somewhat less than twenty-four minutes. Fred's exercise program is more intense—walking or jogging longer distances every day and shaping and toning his muscles using weight machines or isometrics. In 1981, when he was interviewed as background for the case study paper based on his repeat angiogram, he reported that he was running six to eight miles a day and was not experiencing any angina. Fred is leaner than Jack, more streamlined. Both the same age, Jack seems to convey comfortable adaptation with age. His movements are slower and more relaxed than those of Fred, who moves quickly, always at an urgent pace. Says Jack, "I feel my body is changing and I'm waiting a while to see which way it goes before I reestablish my muscle toning exercises."

These days, sports for Jack are mostly of the spectator variety. He holds season tickets to the Lakers and the sport teams of UCLA. Sometimes he uses them; sometimes he gives them to friends. His other diversions are also noncompetitive, including the Philharmonic concerts, his work with retarded children and continued contact with friends and associates from the old days. "We still have a scholarship fund for the high school," he explained to me. "Every year, we get together and give them money." Fred's primary diversion, by his own admission, is work; his relaxation, like our visit to the horse show, is achievement-related. Asked what kind of plans he has for his new son, Fred answered, "I just hope he's happy, just happy," then adding, "healthy, that's all. That's all you can expect—to be healthy and good. I won't push him, I don't want him to emulate me at all."

Traveling provides a sense of self-satisfaction for both men. Jack and his wife, Edie, frequently travel to Mexico City where they have friends, and in fact, during the severe 1985 earthquake in Mexico, Jack kept in contact through his ham radio. "That's why I got it," he explains, "so we can get a hold of them easily." A recent trip to China was so rewarding that Jack says he wants to return again soon. The huge house in Beverly Hills is gone now. Jack and Edie live in a comfortable condominium. Full-time investment counseling doesn't tax a man who is used to running three businesses simultaneously, so Jack uses his excess energy in various volunteer causes and, as he says, in "self-gratification." He reports no physical or psychological complications from his bypass surgery, no health problems at all, in fact. And you can bet that if something came up, he would set himself up to beat it.

Prior to the 1960s, if you were unlucky enough to have developed heart disease, chances are your treatment amounted to little or nothing at all, specifically that you did nothing and aspired to little. The goal was to avoid overtaxing your damaged heart by undue physical activity. Some amount of exercise seemed to be called for in order to strengthen what function remained, but the exact equation was difficult to calculate. So to be on the safe side, the great majority of heart attack victims opted for less than more.

And so developed the lamentable image of the post-heart attack patient slinking around in a life that too often became a mere shadow of its former self. The technological advances that made it possible for Jack Rutta to have the blockage in his coronary arteries bypassed and give him another chance also helped diagnose Fred Rizk's problem and warned him of the risks he was incurring. Two individuals, with two separate approaches to a common problem that affected their lives and the lives of those around them. Two different kinds of courage. Think what it must have meant, for example, for Fred Rizk to defy his doctor's advice and take himself to the unknown regions of the Pritikin center. And also try to appreciate the quiet perseverance of Jack Rutta, who spent the convalescence from his heart attack amusing himself with little tasks around the house instead of dissolving into anger or despair.

Two different men, two diverse types of courage, but one common commitment: To take responsibility for their life and meet its challenges head on. In their stories, there are lessons for all of us.

Chapter 5

Pam Mulhair, 43. Married, no children. Co-owner of Precision Cutting Tools, a metals fabrication plant.

Diagnosis: small vessel disease, leading to two heart attacks and kidney failure.

I

"I think somewhere along the line I finally realized that one of my major mistakes in my life before this—and it was not related just to business—was I do not seem to understand or have any conception of the word moderation in anything. If I do anything, I do it 110 percent. So that makes me the hardest person on me. It's not the people around me. They don't demand from me half of what I demand of myself."

Myths are common beliefs that, although lurking unacknowledged in our everyday lives, give shape to the reality we perceive. They are based on common experience, often the result of our attempts to reduce complicated matters to manageable form. And most myths persist even when challenged by contrary experience; indeed, myths, if they are strong and pervasive enough can function as buffers against reality.

Myths about heart disease would seem to be no different from others that influence our lives. We "know," for example, that men tend to deny serious illness, particularly if the illness is related to the heart. They demonstrate this by falling back into the routines that have obviously contributed to their disease. Men are also "dispassionate" about such ailments, perhaps because this kind of illness strikes at the very core of their virility, inducing a tendency to avoid its implications. Other commonly accepted myths persuade us that men can be slow to take advice about rehabilitation after accident and affliction, and that they may even disregard it completely. On the other hand, the story

148

goes that men face such adversities with more detachment than women because their intellectual coping skills are more developed.

Myths about women and serious illness would suggest that women might respond to such incapacity with emotion and, unlike their male counterparts, be crushed and unable to recover. Or conversely, that women, supposedly more intuitive than men, would turn their intuition in on themselves and squelch potential problems before they arise— even women faced with challenges and pressures similar to what men have been exposed to for years. In this scenario a woman would *sense* when something was not right, and from within her infinite practicality she would initiate steps to alleviate her problem or difficulty.

A review of the statistics on women and heart disease exposes some fallacies in these myths. For example, the rate at which women are experiencing heart disease has increased with their recent influx into the marketplace. Additionally, researchers suggest that in following patterns established by their male front-runners, women expose themselves to the risk factors typically afflicting men: too much pressure, too many business lunches, smoking, excessive alcohol intake and lack of exercise. Most of all, such women court the self-neglect and lack of awareness that characterize the legendary Type A.

Although previously an exclusively all-male club, the Type A behavior pattern has become more noticeable in women. Meyer Friedman and his researchers have determined, for example, that Type A professional women suffer from coronary heart disease almost seven times as frequently as Type B women who remain in the home. Even more revealing, the Framingham study indicates that coronary heart disease is four times more prevalent in employed women who are Type A than in Type B employed women. Friedman and his associates conclude that Type A career women suffer from heart disease just as frequently as the Type A men with whom they work.

Pam Mulhair's story tends to corroborate the statistics, while unraveling simultaneously some of our closely held myths about women. The way she carries herself, the intensity of her speech show her robust disregard for the conventional accoutrements of femininity. But you want to hear in her own words how a woman reacts to this incident called a heart attack, to gain insight, however tentative, into the speculation that women's foray into the supposedly dangerously high-pressure business world might—as the statistics suggest—affect women in the same way it has men, and perhaps most importantly, to determine whether a woman's often finely honed coping skills might aid her in her recuperation. Would she tend to a clearer more realistic self-assessment, and implement needed changes? Are women generating new myths?

You could be overwhelmed by the extent of Pam Mulhair's physical problems. It would not be difficult. She has received the traditional warning signs and ignored them, repeatedly. She has driven the implications of heart disease to the limit. She is truly on the edge of survival. Yet she pushes forward, ever renewing—with an informed optimism that women perhaps can best lay claim to—her efforts to modify her behavior. And yet, some of the Type A pattern is evident: the desire for control, the impulse to be critically involved in the lives of other people. In the power of its implications for both sexes, Pam Mulhair's story is unique. As a study in perseverance and faith, it is an unassuming, provocative rendering of a very personal struggle.

Sitting in her office in one of those faceless suburban industrial parks, Carolyn "Pam" Mulhair, a forty-three-year-old businesswoman who lives and works in Huntington Beach, California, attempts to explain the facts of her continuing struggle with heart disease and its effects. As we talk, Pam, who is dressed in a heavy, baggy red sweater, gray slacks and wedgy sandals, rocks back and forth in her executive chair. Now and then she leans forward and drops her weight on the desk in front of her. Her hands are often busy, fiddling with a paper clip, twisting a rubber band. The mailman comes and offers other opportunities. She takes out a letter opener and begins to open the envelopes one by one, sorting them in neat piles in front of her, all of this while we continue our dialogue. I notice that her only jewelry is a wedding band and a watch with a metal bracelet that slides loosely up and down her left arm.

In answer to my first question about her health, Pam turns her left arm over and traces the outline of a piece of tubing, obvious now, and I understand why the watch is worn loose. She says, "It runs from the scar here . . . about a foot." The graft appears to be about a quarter-inch wide in an elliptical shape running almost from her wrist to her elbow. Caught immediately under the skin, it looks hard and uncomfortable.

I asked if it bothers her, if it inhibits her arm or hand movement.

"No," she answers. "It's just laid in there. They make a track and they lay it under the surface of the skin and they cut and attach it to the artery here and the vein there so that it creates a freeway. It's larger than a blood vessel so it gives a good flow for getting blood through the machine and back into the body again. It's an old system. A lot of people have had terrible problems with their grafts—they clot and they don't last. This is my original graft and I've never had a bit of problem with it."

I know that Pam is no longer on conventional dialysis so I ask if she's ever thought of taking the graft out.

"Oh, no," she answers rapidly, "I would never take it out. It's an insurance policy. I use it fairly frequently anyway, they use it for giving me transfusions or for drawing blood. They do this in the dialysis unit because they say nobody else really knows how to handle the grafts. You see, once you puncture this, if you don't apply the right kind of pressure, you've got a pump that literally just pushes the blood out. I believe that's perhaps what Nathan cut when he committed suicide. I could cut this graft and I'd be dead in probably a matter of twelve minutes.

"With a tiny pin hole it'll pump half a cup a minute. You'd get sleepy and cold and just begin to go away. I know because this is what happens to me when I start losing blood. I get more and more tired as my oxygen-carrying ability drops. Then I start to get angina. It gets harder for me to breathe and everything's a struggle." She drops her voice and sounds like a weak person having difficulty remaining conscious. Her arms hang limp, her shoulders droop in imitation of someone who cannot make one movement further. "Even just getting up and walking across the room takes everything you've got." Her voice drops lower still, fading, as if someone has turned down the volume on a radio.

"The other system works better for me," she continues, "because in the dialysis machine you destroy a certain amount of red blood cells; they get damaged going through the kidneys and the machine and you don't feel as well. You get these peaks and valleys. It's a theory—nobody can prove it—that the PD [peritoneal dialysis] system works so naturally that the body begins to again become levelized, acclimatized; everything starts to function again, almost normally. And it allows the kidneys, if they have anything left at all, to kick in and do a few of their jobs like triggering blood production and some of the things they get lazy and quit trying to do. Because of this a lot of people who have very bad problems with being anemic after a few months on CAPD start building blood again. Their levels come back up and many of them never have to have transfusions again."

Pam, I know, has not been among these lucky people. She requires regular blood transfusions.

"I had one on Tuesday," she says. "I had one the week before on Monday—these are all two units. I went three weeks before that and I had two units. Three weeks before that I had two units. I would guess, and it's just a guess, that I've had approximately 130 units in the last two years. It's Russian roulette, every time I have a unit of blood. You don't know what you're going to get. You don't know if you're going to pick up something really strange. You don't know if you're going to get a type that doesn't quite match. You don't know. They don't know. The medical people can't figure out where my blood's going because they've tested and tested and tested and they can't find a leak.''

Pam's blood loss is unusual. "Out of their entire population over there at the hospital,'' she says, "I'm probably the worst as far as anemia and blood count. Of course mine's aggravated by the fact that I can't tolerate as low a crit [hematocrit level] as some of the other patients, because of my heart. They start to get nervous when I get below twenty-seven. I can make it down now to about twenty-three but when I do, like Tuesday morning, I was just sitting there asleep. I would sit down in the chair and I was gone and I just . . .'' Again the volume fades.

The hematocrit level that Pam speaks of is the ratio of blood cells to liquid plasma. For the normal individual this is usually about forty-five percent. If the body has too few red blood cells, less than say twenty-five to thirty percent, the heart has to pump harder in order to keep oxygen in the tissues. As Pam indicated, also, a low percentage of red blood cells causes weakness and lethargy due to insufficient oxygen. Conversely, if there are too many red blood cells—greater, say, than fifty percent—the blood becomes too thick and also overloads the heart's pumping capacity.

Pam says she can tell when her blood ratios are off and she needs a transfusion. "I can start feeling the fade, and for a while I can keep pushing myself and pushing myself and pushing myself. A lot of times it's just a matter of sheer willpower to force my body to get up and move and keep going. But I don't want blood from any place but St. Mary's in Long Beach. I plan my trips so I never need blood anywhere else.

Pam's GP, Dr. Gerald Anderson, remembers an occasion when she required blood—two units. "It was right after she left the Pritikin center,'' he says. "Her blood count was so low that if it had been mine, I wouldn't have been able to sit up in a chair. Pam insisted, however, that she be transfused in her left hand so she could sit in bed and run an adding machine with her right. Then right after that,'' he concludes with awe in his voice, "she got on a plane and flew to Manila.''

"Would you say,'' I asked Pam, "given everything that's happened to you up to this point, that this mysterious blood loss is perhaps the cause of a real solid fear?''

"Well,'' she answers, "let's say I would be a lot more comfortable from every standpoint if I didn't have to have the amount of transfusions I do. But I still do not have what you'd call a real fear of them. I do know there's probably a possibility that someday I'm going to run into a blood type that I'm going to react to. They're careful about crossing and matching, but they still could miss a little bit too. The risk, I think, is maybe not as great now, because I've had so many that my antibody system is somewhat fooled and it wouldn't be quite as prone to rejection. I literally have no blood of my own left.

"All I can hope is that one of these days we'll find something that makes sense. But if we could stop that, if we could stop the blood loss, I would then be capable of living about an eighty percent normal life." She adds, casually, "Now I figure I am about fifty percent. I automatically now have to figure that I lose one day every three weeks in the clinic because I've got to go get the blood and get the tests. The last two or three days of a three-week period, I'm at forty percent efficiency because I can't move that well . . . I'm slower. I'm running out of gas, I'm running on three cylinders."

She sits and thinks a moment or two. "Besides slowing me down," she says, "it doesn't really keep me from doing much of the things I want. I probably don't travel as much as I would because it does take some planning. It restricts things I would like to be able to do like getting out and swimming and playing a good rough game of beach volley ball. But other than real strenuous exercise or heavy lifting, things that I used to be able to do without thinking, now I at least think about them before I do them."

To my suggestion that she's very dispassionate about her health problems, Pam answers, "Like I say . . . I tend to take things as they come. I don't worry a great deal about them. If it's something I feel I can control, I do. And it's hard for me to really sit down and look at it as an incapacitating illness. When I'm sitting in a hospital bed and I can't get out, I think, 'Gee, maybe it is time for me to think about this,' but on a normal basis, my mind is so occupied all the time with this and that project and things going on, I don't . . . I can't recognize myself as being an invalid or being sick."

The late-winter California sky hangs gray and menacing along the coast south of Los Angeles, striking once and for all any hopes for a sunny weekend. Smog is mixed with the fog, less dense this close to the ocean, but even so there will be few people out this Saturday morning to walk the beaches or ride the bike paths or sit on their boards waiting for the surf. A day like this you sit at the dining room table and catch up on your bills, or restain the antique dresser you picked up last summer or plan the spring garden. Or if you're Pam Mulhair, you go into work.

The flat clouds provide a canopy for the equally flat landscape of this recently developed industrial park about forty miles south of metropolitan Los Angeles. There is nothing outstanding in this new development. The buildings all look the same, flat and low, painted or sprayed gray or white or beige. One guesses there are manufacturing plants and assembly areas that sprawl for portions of acres underneath the crushed-rock roofs.

The Mulhairs' building does little to distinguish itself. A small glass-walled reception area opens into a long hall—executive offices on the street side, doors obviously leading to the manufacturing area on the interior of the building. Pam's office is large and bright. The walls are neutrally beige. The furniture is lightly stained oak with plaid upholstery. A big oak desk sits in the middle of the room, positioned so that its occupant can immediately intercept people coming in the front door and simultaneously converse with anyone sitting in the visitor chairs in front of her.

It's not what you would think of as a woman's office in our modern age of women executives. But then Pam Mulhair was a businesswoman long before many contemporary female executives were out of high school. The office is streamlined and functional, a few pieces of bric-a-brac sit here and there on cluttered surfaces. Some plants recline lazily on a shelf in front of a low window and provide the only real decoration in the room. The window, which runs the length of the office, is almost at floor level, and because the building is raised, the effect is that you look out past a green lawn to the sidewalk. Pam uses the window throughout our conversation, gazing through it past her immediate environment as she pauses, shifting through her recollections, searching for the right anecdote.

Your first impression is that Pam Mulhair doesn't look well. Her skin is pale and pasty and her body is heavy. Then you remember the kidney failure and attribute her complexion to that. Not a drop of makeup relieves the paleness of her face. Her hair is very light, without highlights—another shade from the palette that produced her complexion. If you passed her quickly on the street, you would say this woman is ill, perhaps very ill. She doesn't appear to be overweight, nor is she thin, but her squarely built, large-boned frame gives you the impression of permanency.

Despite initial impressions, something suggests the incongruous opinion that this woman is going to be around for a while. The conclusion is clinched when you focus on her eyes. They provide the only bright spot in her otherwise monochromatic face. They sparkle, they dart, they smile, they laugh, ponder, remember. They are the barometer of her emotions. Her voice is almost consistently strong and steady, whether she is talking about her motor home, her antique furniture collection or reliving her medical experiences. Only occasionally does it drop in reflection or contemplation. She chooses her words easily, clips the final consonants sharply, uses more words than few. She moves with agility; there are no moments of feeble hesitation in this woman's walk.

"Hi there," she says, as I walk toward her office. It's been almost three years since we've seen each other. She was thinner then. Dressed more stylishly. I don't recall the paleness then, the absence of makeup. "How about some breakfast?" she asks. We stand in the hall and exchange pleasantries, like two passengers discovering one another in a narrow hall on a train. The door opens behind me. A tight, muscular man who looks to be in his mid-fifties, swings open the door from the plant side of the hall. Pam introduces us. "This is my husband, Mickey." Mickey answers with a solid handshake and a wary, "Pleased to meet you."

The three of us pile into Pam's dark-green Lincoln Continental for the short ride to the coffee shop. Mickey drives. The restaurant is obviously familiar and both order with only a brief glance at the menu. I drink my decaffeinated coffee and wait. Finally we're settled.

"When did you have your heart attack?" I ask her.

"October, 1978," Pam replies.

"Did you have any idea you had heart problems?"

Mickey answers before Pam, who is still arranging silverware and napkins around the table top. "She had none," he says. And then he adds, as if Pam deliberately forgot to tell him something crucial about their future plans, "I had no idea she was going to have a heart attack."

Pam softens his answer, "I had really been feeling lousy for probably two months before, but I hadn't connected it."

Mickey continues, "One night at the shop she just said she was real tired and wanted to go home about five o'clock. So we went home—we only lived five minutes from the plant—and I had to help her out of the car and up the steps. Then she couldn't move any farther into the house, so I called the paramedics."

Mickey admits it was scary. "Three ambulances came," he says. "They got her to the hospital, and it was a heart attack. Right away I panicked. You know, I knew nothing about the office, the administration. I only know the plant. Pam ran the office."

Pam laughs. "He didn't even know where his bank accounts were."

"I had to borrow money because I didn't know where the accounts were or what was in them. Usually we never saw each other all day. I was downstairs in the plant and she directed the girls in the office.''

"By the time I got to the hospital," Pam continues, "I had had the heart attack. It had probably actually started around three-thirty that afternoon. I had just kind of thought I had indigestion. A close friend of ours and I had gotten one of these earthen crocks, and all summer, while those little pickling cucumbers were out, we had been making pickles. So we always had a batch of pickles going . . ."

Mickey interrupts, "They're gourmet cooks."

"And I had really overdone it," Pam continues. "I had eaten several of them that day and I thought, 'Well, it's indigestion.' But the pain kept getting worse and worse and by the time I had left the shop and gotten home, I had reached a point where I couldn't breathe. And my pressure started to fade so badly that by the time the paramedics got there, I was probably 80 over 50 and dropping." (Normal blood pressure is usually 120 over 80.)

"I hadn't had any symptoms before," she remembers, "nothing to judge by. I had actually felt lousy for about two months before that. Of course," she adds with hindsight, "now I would know that it was a warning sign but at the time I didn't. I didn't connect it."

I asked how bad the heart attack was. Pam answers evenly, "The doctor told my family there was probably a good chance I wouldn't get through the night. You see, I made it through the initial part of the heart attack OK. I was taken in about six-thirty in the evening and it seemed to level off, and of course as soon as they gave me the morphine, the pain subsided. It wasn't so much pain actually as the unpleasant pressure of not being able to breathe. That was the really the worst problem. I felt like a tremendous weight was sitting on me." She pauses for a sip of coffee. "But the most frightening thing was that I started having PVCs [premature ventricular contractions occurring in the area of Pam's heart that pumps blood to the body; the result is an irregular heartbeat], which I'm prone to and have had for many many years. They were getting horrible, however, like fifteen a minute. This interrupted the heart rhythm so badly that the doctors figured it was their biggest problem. So they put me on a lidocaine drip and it took them four or five hours until they could get the irregularities to level out and get a normal heart rate again. The cardiologist remembers that as really his worst time. The PVCs started about midnight, so apparently this was a result of the damage the heart had suffered."

A number of factors can influence an irregular heart beat, including emotional stress and deprivation of oxygen. During a heart attack, however, the normal function of the heart's muscle cells is disrupted and the cells begin to work in an irregular fashion. So in Pam's case, the fibrillation, as medicine calls this phenomenon, was a result of a loss of oxygen caused by her heart attack.

Setting down his coffee cup, Mickey picks up the story. He explains that while Pam was in the hospital for two weeks he tried to hold the business together. "I worried a lot," he says. " 'Course I had some good people at the plant. We had a couple of sisters working for us, so it ran all right."

Pam adds her two cents, "He smoked a lot."

"And then it got so Pam was running the place from her bed."

"Yep," she says. "By the second or third day, as soon as I could get the telephone situation straightened out, I was back doing business again." But while Pam acted like it was business as usual, Mickey says he knew they would have to sell the plant and began to look for a buyer.

"When I left the hospital," Pam says, "they gave me the basic American Heart Association diet and put me on a rehab and exercise program and I did pretty well for six or eight weeks. Then, of course, once I could begin to sneak back over to the shop a little, I went back to my old habits. Back to working too many hours and being there too long.

"That," she laughs, "is when Mickey said, 'It's got to go.' But I wasn't happy at all about the whole thing. I didn't see it that way. I didn't see that the plant had anything to do with anything else. Although it was ultimately a very good move, to me at the time selling the plant was like taking away something that was mine. And when you've spent that many hours and that many years building something, you don't want to just give it up."

Mickey remembers the day of the sale. "We were upstairs with all the attorneys and accountants and everything. We were signing our stock over to them and they were giving us their stock. Pam was crying—she never cries—she was crying like a baby. God . . ."

"I just kept thinking, 'My company is going," says Pam.

"Later," Mickey responds, "I thought it was like selling your kid."

"It was," says Pam.

"Or like selling your dog."

"No," she says, "it was like selling my kid."

"It took a long time to get over that."

The business the Mulhairs speak of so fondly is not a glamour business. Nor is it the kind of business commonly associated with contemporary women executives, a service industry or consumer-oriented business. Precision Cutting Tools grew out of Mickey's aptitude for designing and building industrial machinery to fabricate parts for heavy industry. The bulk of their business is with companies such as Rocketdyne International. The Mulhairs have been the sole owners of their operations, financing their efforts with their own capital and investments.

It's a fiercely independent life-style. They have carved a niche for themselves and serve their customers well. Both Mickey and Pam are well-grounded in the old-style American work ethic. Explains Mickey, "If I say I can make a machine, I do it right. I don't fool around. Quality and service, that's what counts." Both feel their integrity and capacity for hard work have afforded them not only the opportunity to be financially successful but to live the type of life-style they enjoy. "Working for someone else," says Pam, "is very difficult, especially when you've always been your own boss."

And although the Mulhairs have available to them numerous recreational opportunities—two houses, one of which is at the beach, a large motor home, a vacation house in the Colorado desert—work is the cornerstone of their life. Nine-to-five appears not to be in either's vocabulary. Says Pam, "I get up sometimes on Friday mornings and I say, 'Gee, only one more day this week. I can't get everything done I need to do. I need two more days this week.' It's a challenge and it's fun and it's never boring."

Mickey remembers the sale of their first company with some bitterness. "They romanced us into believing that everything was going to be handled well and then they turned right around and ran it into the ground. It didn't even take them a year."

"That," reveals Pam with a flourish, "is when we bought the motor home." She pauses a moment for a bite of her breakfast. "And before it was ready, Mickey had his heart attack." She goes on to explain. "We ordered the thing in February and the dealer called me up in late March and said, 'The mobile home's here.' But Mickey's doctor said he couldn't drive, so I decided this was the time to learn how to drive the bus.

"When Mickey had his attack," she recalls flatly, "I wasn't really worried because I knew that basically he didn't have a cholesterol problem. I knew this was stress, strictly stress overload from watching them destroy what we'd built. It wasn't easy. I just finally walked out of it and shut my eyes and said, 'I won't let it get to me.' But he lets things get to him differently than I do."

Mickey objects, "Normally I don't."

"He's pretty noisy about his stress," Pam continues, "and he gets a lot of it out, but I don't. Mine sort of just sits there and simmers, you know. As the old saying goes, I guess, I don't get mad, I just get even. And that's worse because your mind is always working on it.

"You know," she speculates randomly, "I think any business is a strain. The one we have now has been a lot easier for me because I've changed a lot in the last five years. I take things a lot more in stride. But I had fifteen years of blood, sweat and tears wrapped up into that first company. We've only worked on this one for two-and-a-half years and already it's the same size the other one was when we sold it. But with this one I've got an arm's-length deal in my own mind."

"Yeah," agrees Mickey, "it will run without us."

Pam Mulhair says she's been working for thirty years, and you tend not to doubt her. Born in the Midwest, she's been married to Mickey for twenty-eight years, since she was fifteen, and the two of them have been in business together throughout their marriage. Pam's sister died of ovarian cancer in 1980, and a younger brother lives in Idaho. Careful study of her heredity might have provided clues about the medical challenges she would eventually face. One of Pam's maternal aunts, for example, suffered from diabetes, another from diabetes and heart problems. A third had severe kidney problems. Still another aunt had been blind from early age, possibly the result of juvenile-onset diabetes. One of these women lived to be eighty—with severe kidney and abdominal problems—and another to her early sixties even with diabetes and heart-related illness. Pam's mother is in her eighties and until recently lived alone in Oregon; her father died of a stroke at seventy-one. An uncle suffered from high cholesterol and died of a heart attack at age seventy-six.

Pam's vision of her heredity is fatalistic. "Well, you think about everything," she says. "But with heredity there's not a lot you can do but look at patterns for road maps. I mean, sure you can look at it and say, 'I'm doomed, what the hell, it doesn't matter anyhow.' But I look at life a little differently. I feel like, well, I'm definitely not ready to go. I don't have everything done yet, and I just somehow have a feeling that I have a good many years yet." She pauses and begins to express another thought. "Anyhow," she says, "my fear is not dropping dead . . ." Her voice lowers here, becoming almost soft. "My fear is becoming incapacitated. That's the only fear I have. And strangely enough with all of these other things that have happened to me, if I have a fear at all, it is of blindness."

She stops, lets that sink in. "Because I don't know that I could face life blind." She pauses again, turns in her chair and looks off in the distance. "I think so long as I've got my mental facilities and my eyes, I can make it.'' Then the thought brightens. ''You know what I mean, especially in today's world—with the gadgets. We can run the world from a room.

''So,'' she concludes, ''probably the only thing I'm really faithful about is getting my eye checkup, and fortunately—she raps her knuckles on the wood of her desk—''there appears to have been no diabetic damage at all.''

After her heart attack, Pam didn't spend much time evaluating the life-style that might have contributed to it. ''I'll admit,'' she says, ''that heart attack didn't really get my attention as much as it should have, even though I really didn't feel real good again until October. Everybody yelled at me. None of the family would let anybody at the shop talk to me. If they wanted to talk to me, they had to sneak out and call me at home.

''You see,'' she explains with a suggestion of self-mockery in her voice, ''I do excessive things. If something tastes good, it wouldn't be enough for me to have a half a glass of it or whatever; I'd have to drink the whole thing. I used to do this. I'd sit down and drink a half gallon of buttermilk at a time. I'd drink a half gallon of sweet milk at a time. Now, when I think about the amount of cholesterol in the cheeses and milk . . .'' The thought ceases, she selects another. ''I used to think I hadn't lived unless I had at least two eggs in a day, sometimes it was even four or five. A lot of times I'd have an omelet or eggs for dinner as well as for breakfast. Too much red meat. I figured I had to have red meat once a day at least. I came from farm country and that's the way you were fed. But when you're flying a desk and trying to eat like a farmer, it doesn't work.''

She clarifies. ''The doctors told me a little about diet and exercise after the first attack, but I didn't pay much attention to it. I tried to quit smoking, which was very frustrating because I was a very heavy smoker. Food had to become a substitute, because I was still going like this inside—'' She imitates a churning motion with her hands. ''When I had my first heart attack I was smoking three packs a day and probably drinking twenty cups of coffee a day. In fact that was my basic diet, coffee and cigarettes—adrenaline—and I ate anything and everything. I mean I always had a high profile diet as far as red meats and starches and that sort of thing. The only thing I was pretty good about was sweets. We ate out a lot and there was a lot of fast food, quick sandwiches and that sort of thing. While I liked everything and I would eat vegetables and fruits and whatever, I still had a lot of starch and rich sauces and gravies. That's the way my tastes sort of ran.''

Little by little, we begin to dissect Pam's medical history. It is loaded, unfortunately, with a number of highly interrelated factors that eventually accumulated in the showdown of a heart attack in 1978 at the age of thirty-six. Although she maintains the heart attack came as a surprise, she acknowledges an awareness of her high cholesterol level.

"I have always known I had a cholesterol problem. I would guess that probably as early as 1970 or '71, my cholesterol count would run normally anywhere between 400 and 600," she says dispassionately. "They put me on everything they could think of—the cholesterol blockers, the cholesterol reducers. But quite honestly," she concludes, "I have come to believe throughout the years that my body literally produces cholesterol and that it doesn't have a whole lot to do with my diet. A friend of mine is the same way. We've been close for about twenty years and we've sort of been through some weird medical things together. He has very severe leg blockage, even though he's been real careful about his diet. I mean fanatically careful. But it doesn't really seem to make much difference. His cholesterol levels remain the same. I've decided that it has something to do with stress patterns—his temperament is very much like mine. If you run on high octane, maybe the body thinks it needs this extra cholesterol for some reason. He comes from a fairly large family of six or eight children and they've all come up with some sort of a cholesterol-related problem. So that kind of brings it back to the question of, is it hereditary? Is there something in the genes that helps cause it or at least allows it to happen?"

I asked Pam if she had an angiogram after her first heart attack. "Yes, in November of 1978," she says. "They found two fairly severe blockages and one moderate one, but the blockages are not in the main aorta areas. They're all inside the heart in the smaller veins that actually feed the feeders. That's why I'm not even a bypass candidate."

Mickey adds another clarification, "That's why they won't give her a kidney transplant—because of her heart."

"Well . . ." Pam continues, as if she might dispute what Mickey says, but lets it go. "There are two areas of feeder veins that had eighty percent blockage and one area that had about fifty percent. My doctor felt that not much of that could be reversed, but if we could knock the cholesterol levels down and get me on a decent exercise program, it might help. He felt that the feeders being small, they might even develop new feeders—collateral circulation. And like I said, I'd been doing pretty well for a while on the exercise and kind of watching myself. Then I fell off the wagon and started smoking again and going back to work."

The "feeders" Pam refers to are the small blood vessels that help supply blood to the heart, branching off the three main coronary arteries. The diagnosis of Pam's condition at the time was what is called small vessel disease, probably a result of the diabetes she also suffered from. Her physician, Dr. Anderson, explains: "Due to a rapid onset of diabetes," he says, "Pam developed small vessel disease, which affects primarily the tiny arteries in the kidneys, eyes and brain. It's not as significant in the heart." Individuals with diabetes, however, also tend to run high cholesterol levels, which can lead to atherosclerosis, the accumulation of plaques in the arteries of the body. So, in effect, Pam suffered from two types of circulatory problems—the small vessel disease that affected her kidneys as well as her heart, and atherosclerosis in her larger arteries.

Listening to his wife's quiet recitation of her medical problems and the life-style that she acknowledges probably contributed to them, Mickey Mulhair interrupts with an important clarification. "But we couldn't have stayed together," he explains, "if Pam had been just a housewife. Because while she's in the shop until nine at night, I'm down there working on my things."

Mickey Mulhair is about ten years older than his wife. Except for a hint of excess pounds at his waist, he is thin and muscular, and unlike Pam, small-boned. He seems to share her irreverence for style and dresses for comfort and practicality. Your first impression is that he'd be a hard man to beat, that he's tough and opinionated. His opinions are characterized by a clear simplicity of thought that serves him well. He does not, however, appear to be the type of man who'd select a career woman for his wife. Nonetheless, Pam supports his contention about the ties that bind their relationship. "We understand the passions that we both have for the business," she offers. "And I think a great deal of the cement of our relationship is the fact that we have so much in common as far as working habits, and most of our outside interests are the same."

That fact established, and slowly changing the subject, Pam concludes, "Now you get an idea of what happened to me, when after my heart attack, Mickey told me we were going to sell the business and retire. I went home and went like this." She drums her fingers along the table top.

"That's why," says Mickey, "I bought the motor home."

"And later that year after he'd recovered from his heart attack," Pam continues, "in mid-June, we decided we'd take a trip up to the Pacific Northwest because we both have a lot of relatives up there. So we left here and took two of Mickey's sisters and just wandered up along the coast. By July we were crossing the Columbia River on our way to Spokane to see his aunt. We were driving along pretty uneventfully and then about three o'clock one afternoon I started to not feel too well.

"I was quiet about it," she says, continuing the narrative, "but my two sisters-in-law were watching, and along about seven o'clock in the evening, one of them decided she would try to feed me. Her cure for everything is to feed you. If you can eat, you're going to make it. But I just couldn't do it. I just couldn't get anything down. Mickey's other sister noticed, however, that my face was becoming an ashen color. Finally I told them I was going to lie down. They left me alone for a while and then one of them came back and switched on the light and saw that, by that time, my lips were blue. She asked me how I felt. I told her I really didn't feel good. For me to even make a comment like that, they knew it was time to look for someone."

"So," says Mickey, "I'm going about eighty or ninety miles an hour to the hospital . . ."

But Pam is determined to tell the story and interrupts him. "At that point we were just outside a little town called Othello, Washington, with no hospital, no doctor, no nothing. We had to go to the next town, where there was a little hospital but they had no doctor. They were serviced by a paramedic. So they hooked me into the heart center in Spokane while the nurse called the paramedic, who lived just out of town, I guess. When he arrived, the first thing he said was, 'We've got to make her comfortable and start helping her to relax, so I'm going to give her a shot of morphine.' This was about eight o'clock in the evening. After that he got on the phone with Spokane trying to make arrangements for the heart unit to come out and get me by air ambulance. But the helicopter was tied up with a blue baby emergency somewhere else. I told him I thought I could wait for a surface ambulance to come and get me. But he still worried about me being uncomfortable, so he decided to give me another shot of morphine at midnight. At two-thirty, he must have thought I might be having some more pain, so he gave me another shot of morphine."

Mickey interrupts, with the first of his many classic one-liners, "Damn near killed her."

Pam continues. "Finally about three-thirty or four in the morning, the heart unit got there and they checked me out and got me hooked up to their equipment in the van and got ready to leave with me. The paramedic said, 'I've got to make sure that she feels OK for the trip,' and gave me another morphine shot at five o'clock.

"But by this time," she remembers, "it was pouring rain—one of the worst storms I've ever seen in my life, and the ambulance was driving 110 miles an hour down these wet roads."

"It was spooky as hell," says Mickey. "I was driving the motor home. They got to town about two hours before me."

Pam concludes the story of her ride to the hospital. "About halfway to town, my hair started to itch and tingle. I must have been having a horrible reaction to the morphine. Finally they got me into town about seven o'clock in the morning. They rolled me into the heart ward, and I must have vomited for about twenty minutes, which dehydrated me completely. My body was trying to get rid of all that morphine. I said, 'If anybody ever tries to come near me again with a needle, I'm going to kill them.' "

Mickey sits quietly and listens. He has not yet eaten much of his breakfast. Pam goes on to describe how she felt when she finally arrived at the hospital. "Once I got through all that trauma, I felt OK. It wasn't like the time before. I didn't feel tired and worn out, although it did leave me with more heart damage. The doctor up there decided that he would put me on aspirin, which interrupts the platelet action enough to inhibit blood clots. So he put me on twenty grains of aspirin a day."

Mickey interjects, "Damn near ate her stomach up."

"Well," says Pam, "then I came back down here and talked to my cardiologist and he said that aspirin was a good idea, that it was one of the best and safest blood thinners. So I figured, 'Well, all right.' "

A bit amazed at her capacity for self-punishment, I asked Pam Mulhair if she continued smoking and maintained her work schedule after the second attack.

"Yes," she replies thickly. "Stupid is the word for it."

II

"The thing is that money itself isn't important to me, but it's a good way to keep score. You can tell by looking at my bank account if I'm playing the game right."

Many people who work long hours in the service of their own business do so partly to enjoy the luxuries their money can buy. You sense this in their surroundings, the way they dress, how they spend their leisure time. The Mulhairs, however, appear to have developed some unique standards by which to measure their success. Pam explains.

"I don't know," she says. "Things like diamonds and furs and Rolls-Royces and all don't interest me. If I've got some money, I'll sit around and I'll look at it for a while, and then I'll think, 'Well, gee, I can buy a couple more machines, and I know they're good investments; they'll make me money,' instead of saying, 'I have all this extra money and I can buy a Rolls-Royce.' ''

"So after a while," says Mickey, "a year or so later, I got a business going, the same type of business we used to have, and then she started butting into that. She had taken a two-month trip in the motor home with my sister and I stayed home working on my racing cars." He looks annoyed. "I figured they'd be poking around looking under every rock, like the two dumb broads they are." Mickey and Pam both laugh. "But soon," he says, "I was getting busier and busier and she was getting more and more involved. She was taking care of the money again."

"I don't know," Pam interrrupts. "I think maybe it would be better for me if maybe I were a little more frightened by the things that have happened to me, but I must have a real funny attitude toward . . ." She pauses a couple of beats and wraps up the thought, "I mean I don't have any terrible fear of dying." She drops the statement casually and before you can assess its implications, Mickey says, "I feel the same way about her. I figure she may go tomorrow but I wouldn't change my life-style. I don't change the way I talk to her or the way I do things. We do the same things we'd do if she were totally healthy."

Pam is silent, appearing to confirm an unwritten agreement between them. "I think what he's trying to say," she starts, "is if someone worried about every little thing with me, they'd be . . ." She stops, interrupting herself, streamlining the sentiment. "There's always something happening to me, but I try, number one, not to let it interfere with the normal day-to-day living. I don't say, 'Oh, I'm an invalid; I can't do these things.''

I venture that a lot of people in her situation would do just that.

"Yeah," she answers, "they'd just sit down and quit, but you see what would happen to them? They wouldn't be here.

"My health problems go way back," she discloses, as the true picture begins to emerge. "The diabetes started abut the same time the high blood pressure kicked in, and the high cholesterol level. My doctor tried for years and years and years to figure out how to control these various things. Like my blood pressure—I was on medication four times a day and my blood pressure was still running 160 over 90; it was just like my engine was in rev all the time. As early as 1970, my cholesterol level was very high, over 600. In early '70, I broke my leg and was in the hospital for a couple of weeks. I had this humongous cast on but the fracture wouldn't heal. I was in the cast from February of 1970 to January of '71—eleven months." She pauses and adds, "The doctors were of course curious as to why I wasn't healing. That's when they found excessive blood-sugar levels and the high blood pressure."

You catch your breath at all of this and shudder at its potential accumulated effects. Facts flash forward. Medicine has identified that women with diabetes run three times the normal risk of developing heart disease. And although female hormones are thought to help reduce heart disease risk, diabetes (and the use of oral contraceptives) can negate their positive effects. And the diuretics frequently prescribed for high blood pressure can affect the body's potassium level, which is related to kidney function, and can also disturb the normal rhythm of the heart. High blood pressure, suffered by some 38 million Americans, can also be symptomatic of kidney abnormality. The Framingham study reported that women with high blood pressure—defined as 160/95 or higher— had three times the risk of coronary artery disease that those with the normal blood pressure of 120/80 did. The Framingham study also reported that in women it has followed between the ages of forty and fifty, high cholesterol (260 or better) triples the risk of heart disease. Pam Mulhair seemed to be flirting with a time bomb.

"In 1973," Pam continues, "they put me on oral medication for the diabetes and told me something about diet. That's when I learned to cut out all the desserts and sugars. I did break that habit, thank goodness. Then," she says, "another thing happened in 1973." This time the remembrance is positive. "I decided I wanted to get my pilot's license. So when I went to get my medical clearance, I filled out the medical information form completely, with all the medications I was taking. Obviously they disqualified me." She laughs, "They didn't want me in the sky. So," she discloses, as if it were inevitable, "I had my big run-in with the FAA physician and asked him how I was going to be able to get a medical clearance. He said, 'When you take off some weight, when you control your diabetes and blood pressure with diet and you are taking no medications, come and talk to me.' So I went home and lost fifty pounds and got off all my medications. I had everything under control with diet and then went down and got my medical approval.

"Carlton Fredericks' [Pam might have read *Low Blood Sugar and You*] carbohydrate diet controlled my diabetes and hypertension beautifully. My values came right back into normal range. And I felt so much better with the extra weight off. I was exercising, mostly walking, some bicycling."

Although her initial success with modifying her diet sounds like the beginning of a positive trend, things weren't to last. "After I got my license, things really started getting busy for me at the shop because we were in a tough growth pattern. This was probably '74 by then, and health-wise I was not terribly off kilter. The only thing I can remember at that time was that I had a lot of problems with PVCs and they put me on medication to help control them. But I knew,'' she admits passively, "that the heart irregularities were aggravated by the stress, the coffee and the smoking.''

When I ask why she didn't give up coffee or the smoking to help control her blood pressure, she looked at me with a grin. "I wasn't going to do anything that rash,'' she concedes and then continues. "But I went along OK then until early '78 when I began to feel lousy and had the heart attack. In November when I had the first angiogram done, they found a tumor on the right side of my thyroid, so they removed that in December. Then I had the second heart attack in July of '79. In late April of '81, I was admitted to the hospital with what I thought was a kidney stone or a kidney infection. They did a series of studies and they decided it was gallstones.

"By that time,'' she remembers, "I had fallen off the wagon and had put back on quite a bit of weight. Also at that point they noticed there was a slight increase in my creatinine level.'' (Creatinine is a nitrogen compound—one of the wastes eliminated by the kidneys—the measurement of which is used to help determine kidney function. A high creatinine level might, for example, be symptomatic of a dysfunction of the kidneys.) "Even back then,'' she confides, "this was probably a slight indication that the kidneys were getting edgy. That was in April. They told me at that time about diet in relation to gallstones, emphasizing the spicy foods and things that would irritate it. That's when I really started to think seriously about Pritikin. I thought, 'Well, maybe I can really clean up my act.' ''

I asked what made her think of Pritikin.

"I was not overly concerned,'' she explains, "about the weight and the other problems, but I knew I wasn't feeling as good as I should and in fact I was feeling worse and worse. So I thought, 'Well, really, if you've got any intelligence at all, which you claim to have, you'd better clean up your act.' So I decided in February of '81 that I would quit smoking, seriously. Just quit. This was complicated by the fact that in late 1980, we discovered my sister had cancer. I had gone through surgery with her in November but I kind of realized at Christmastime that she had given up. Her husband and I really fought and fought and fought, but eventually by the end of February, she decided to quit chemotherapy. I think that was the toughest psychological battle I've ever been through. Here I was trying to quit smoking, which had always been my psychological crutch.'' She pauses and takes a deep breath to catch up with herself. ''My sister's basically last wish was that she not have to be in the hospital for her last days, but there was just no way she could be alone. So I went to stay with her in Oregon. That was a tough one. I was there from the fourteenth of March and she passed away April 1. But I figured if I made it through that without smoking, I could do anything.''

The waitress comes over and clears the table, providing a short break and Pam a platform from which to spring forward with the rest of her story. ''So having basically survived that,'' she sighs, ''I decided I might just as well keep at it. By that time I had all but quit drinking coffee. I'd have a cup of decaf once in a while, but coffee and cigarettes sort of seem to go together so without one you really didn't need the other. Also, I had this very close friend, my family doctor [Dr. Anderson]. Every time I saw him, he would tell me about this Pritikin Program that he'd been reading about. He kept bugging me, telling me, 'You know, I don't think it would hurt you to try this program.' One day I went in and he had bought the book for me. He gave it to me and said. 'Why don't you just try a modified diet?' '' She pauses and adds the paren-thetical comment, ''I had been going to him since about 1965, and he could see the signposts. I had a lot of albumin in my urine, protein spill, and he could see that could mean some kidney damage or problems. He was real impressed with Nathan's theory about diet. So he said, 'It won't hurt you. Why don't you try it?' ''

Thus on the advice of Dr. Anderson, who was concerned about Pam's constant battle with weight control and hoped the Pritikin Pro-gram would help her make a long-term change in her life-style, Pam decided she might give the program a try. She read the book he had provided for her. When I asked what she thought, she answers glibly, ''I thought, 'This guy's out of his mind. You can't eat like this,' especially since it was such a radical departure from what I was used to doing. But my doctor had asked me to just give it a try, so I messed around a little bit with it.

''From everything I had read,'' she continues, ''it made sense, but it seemed there was such a variety of things that affected cholesterol levels. I knew I was a terrible saltaholic, which I'm sure contributed to the blood pressure, retention of water, fluid in the tissues. Somebody gave me a health questionnaire once. There were nine questions, and six of the risk factors applied to me—like smoking and coffee consumption, the stress, family heredity, long hours and hard work, everything that would contribute . . . I fit the pattern.''

Listening to Pam Mulhair recite the litany of her ailments, you wonder that her body agreed to function. Medicine lumps the composite of her ailments—high blood pressure, diabetes, heart disease—under the comprehensive heading degenerative disease, illness that causes the breakdown of bodily functions and is related to habits of our modern life-style—rich food, lack of exercise. Her high blood pressure alone was a significant risk factor for heart disease. Medical facts indicate, for example, that one out of every six patients suffering from heart disease also has hypertension, and two-thirds of individuals with hypertension die of coronary problems. High blood pressure increases the severity of atherosclerosis because it makes the arteries more permeable to fat, thus actually helping initiate the disease. In fact, it's generally considered that if left untreated, high blood pressure can shorten a person's life by an average of twenty years.

Suffering from three major degenerative diseases, Pam is a classic example of self-neglect, an attitude men have flirted with—and suffered from—for years. One wonders why any one of these problems didn't give her pause to stop and wonder. In this vein, it's interesting to note her opinion that her physician's concern for her is related to his own bad habits. "He rides himself," she says, "a lot like I do—at 110."

Taking her doctor's advice, however, Pam did read a Pritikin book and decided, she says, that "it had some good basic background and theory. I went back over to talk to my doctor and asked him what he thought. Should I just go whole hog and try it? He told me, 'Well, it's not going to hurt you any.' He's one of those people who firmly believes you should implement a program of prevention rather than fix it later, and he thought that maybe the information I could bring back would help him with other patients.

"So I sent in my application to Pritikin. They sent it back and said, 'In light of your history, we don't want you.' They objected to everything," she explains, "but I think the thing they singled out was the heart problem. So we haggled a little bit and they said they would accept me if I had another angiogram and if my doctor felt that I would not be a problem."

Pam says the request for another angiogram didn't bother her. "I figured they were using good common sense. And it really was good news in a way," she says. "I was at least almost holding my own. The cardiologist who did it felt that I would definitely benefit from the diet as well as the exercise program. So I said 'OK' and I was accepted for the early August starting class.

"Mickey came down in the evenings to visit," she remembers. His opinion was that it was a '$6,000 joke' but if I wanted to do it, I should do it. He wasn't real impressed, but then he isn't by most things like that. But I really thought there was a sound basis for this whole thing, and when I went through the indoctrination and introductory presentation, I was really impressed. I thought, 'Somebody's done a lot of research; they have a lot of logical theory here.' "

To my question of how she found the food, she answers blithely, "I didn't care. I'm a salad freak. I could live on salads for a good bit of time. I missed meat, but by that time I had cut down a lot on the red meats myself, trying primarily to eat fish, turkey and chicken." She grins. "I'll admit it was real nice on Thursday night when we did get our one-and-a-half ounce of protein. Everybody was in the dining room fighting over their little bit of meat. But I have to admit, it was real, real good.

"My only problem was that at about the beginning of the third week, I had the most terrible craving. I can't even explain to you how bad. I would have literally given my eye teeth for cottage cheese. Now, why cottage cheese I don't know. At first I thought maybe it was because I'm such a milk and dairy product fanatic. I may have needed the calcium. Then I realized later that normal, prepared cottage cheese has a lot of salt, and I just was craving salt. Here I am, a saltaholic, stuck for two weeks with no salt. Even if you pour all the Tabasco and all the other stuff they give you on your food, it still doesn't take the place of the salt."

She thinks a moment, as if she's remembering something important. "But I did begin to learn to eat a lot of foods and to appreciate the taste of certain foods without salt. Before I went to Pritikin, I salted any kind of starch. I've even been known to put salt on my bread—you know, put butter on it and add salt. I put salt in buttermilk; I put salt on cantaloupe, salt on grapefuit, salt on oranges, salt on apples. I don't think I ate anything without salt. One of the tricks I discovered real quick at the center was that one of the replacements for salt is lemon; you can put lemon on things like baked potatoes." She laughs as she continues. "They'd give us a baked potato and I'd think, 'How do you eat a baked potato without salt and sour cream? Ugh.' Then somebody said to me the second or third day I'd been there, 'You know if you put some fresh lemon juice and a little pepper on it, it's not too bad.' I said, 'Well, I'll try.' I was starving. They told me I should lose a couple of pounds of week, but getting off the salt and still on the diuretics I lost twenty pounds in two weeks. Then she says offhandedly, "And by then the fainting began."

When I asked about the staff's opinion of her cholesterol level, which hadn't dropped as low as she had hoped, Pam answers, "Nathan sort of agreed with me that there were a lot of mysterious question marks in my medical history—and that my medical profile had gotten progressively worse over the years. It almost seems like my system acts exactly the reverse of how it's supposed to work. The cholesterol levels, for instance. I don't think there was anyone in my entire group, my entire class, whose levels didn't drop dramatically in the first three or four or five days. And by the time they were there three weeks, they had wonderful levels. I think mine went down by a factor of 100 and then I think it went back up.

"This was frustrating to the staff at the center. They didn't know how to handle it. In the meantime, my doctor there was beginning to discover all these other little disasters. Finally he decided to do an entire blood panel on me. He took me off the diuretics and pumped me full of potassium and that leveled me right back out. I also had obviously rising creatinine levels, so in the beginning of the third week, they sent me out to see a nephrologist, who confirmed that I had some kidney problems. Everyone hoped it was just a one-time result of the potassium drop and that the kidney function would return to normal. My creatinine levels did begin to go down. Then they realized that I was having trouble with my blood. So they started testing my stool and they discovered that my stomach lining was bleeding from all the aspirin. So immediately they took me off the aspirin and the bleeding stopped."

I wanted to know if any of this made her uncomfortable.

"No," she answers, "even with the hemoglobin drop like that, I didn't really feel it that badly. I felt like I had enough energy and go. My doctor at the center, however, was real concerned about all of the problems collectively and wanted me to be followed up by a nephrologist when I got out. When I left the center, I went back to my original doctor and my Pritikin doctor sent him a volume of reports on me, mostly saying that things looked real good. My kidney function began to reverse and go back to normal." (Dr. Anderson recalls that he spoke about twice a week with the doctor who was following Pam at the center, and he says, "Her doctor there took a real interest in her case.")

"At the center, exercise-wise," Pam explains, "they didn't push me excessively. They gave me a very moderate beginning program for a treadmill and for walking. My first was the lap between the building and down to the pier [a distance of about four-tenths of a mile]. See, it wasn't my chest or my heart that bothered me, it was my legs. My legs would be the first thing that would go. The muscles would cramp and I'd have to stop . . . but the recovery was pretty fast and I was going pretty good on my exercise program until I started having those other problems. Because of all that, they took me off the exercise program, period. After I got home, I tried getting on a routine of walking, starting with half-mile laps.''

"The blood wasn't getting out of your legs?" I asked.

"That's right," she says. "It wasn't being pumped back sufficiently. I do much, much better now. Their theory is that if you keep working at it and working at it and working at it, you do increase your capacity. I think to some degree that's probably what's happened, and especially with the legs, because I can walk probably twice or three times the distance now that I could then.''

Pam remembers that many people at the center—and people in general—couldn't understand how she could be so optimistic and so happy, given her health problems. "I'd tell them," she says with a faint smile, " 'Well, I'm here, I got up this morning and I didn't find my name in the obituary column, so life must be on.' A lot of them didn't understand my feelings. They had had maybe a mild heart attack or had some warnings and were terrified. Actually I found that the ones who were most terrified were those who were facing diagnostic testing, things like an angiogram.

"There were quite a lot of people at the center," she explains thoughtfully, "who literally believed they were invalids. Quite a few of them had experienced much more minor heart attacks than I had, but they were afraid of everything. They were afraid to get up and walk across the room. They were afraid to walk across the street. They couldn't plan a trip because, God forbid, something might happen to them. Their lives had all but stopped.

"It was a challenge," she contends, "because I felt, if I could get a message across to any of them, that it may not be the quantity of life but strictly the quality of life that you have while you're here that's important. And that whatever time they had left should be good and productive and enjoyable instead of being a chore. A lot of them seemed to be making it a chore. They were saying 'Oh, I can't; I can't, I can't.' I'd say, 'You can! You can!' "

I asked Pam if she had had any fear of the angiogram. Unlike men, who most often express no concern about undergoing such diagnostic testing, Pam says, "Yes, especially the first one. More than anything else, it was the fear of the unknown. You've not done it before. You don't know really what it's going to be. I think the thought crossed my mind that I literally could die on the table while they were doing it.''

And again unlike most men, who tend to characterize the procedure as just one in a series of tests, Pam attempted to personalize the experience. "The man who did mine was a young Oriental doctor from UCLA, and I've got to admit I have never seen anything as slick in my life. He talked me through the whole thing and explained to me what was going on—and when the dye was being injected and how to follow it on the screen. There was just nothing to it.

"You know," she proposes, finishing the last cup of decaffeinated coffee, "I think an illness or a problem or a handicap of any kind is basically as major or as minor as you allow it to be. Take two people who have no physical handicaps. One of them gets up every morning, goes to work, or has a project, things that he or she does. They're really biting the bullet, getting every minute out of life. They're communicating and interacting with other people. And maybe the second person lives next door and can't get out of bed till noon, can't get out even to the grocery store till five o'clock, can't move, doesn't interact well, has—whatever the case may be—low self-esteem. He or she doesn't know how to get involved, how to get interested. If you now give the same medical problem to these two people, that first person is going to handle it, and there's going to be no problem. The second person is probably going to lie down and die. Because the motivation wasn't there to begin with."

On that note, Mickey suggests we return to the plant. He has things to do and he's getting impatient with our talk. As he leaves the table to pay the check, Pam continues her thought. "So I think a lot of it is in your mental attitude. You have to either handle it or it handles you. I've been physically at the bottom of the pit several times, and I realized that there are times when the physical problems became so insurmountable, when you just can't mentally force your body to get up and move anymore. It's just physically impossible. Even people who have a strong will like I do have days where they think, 'I wonder if it's really worth the effort to keep pushing. Maybe I should just relax and let whatever happens happen.' And I can do that for about two hours and then . . . you know, it's just not my nature. They're probably going to be closing the lid on my casket and I'm going to be saying, 'Wait a minute, guys. I'm not finished. I've got two more hours of work to do.'" We both laugh, but the image seems entirely probable.

"When I came home from the center," Pam describes, "I started following the Pritikin diet, not to a T, but not even as liberal as the Maintenance Diet. I got myself a box and I went *wh-i-s-s-s-h* with every bit of canned goods and everything processed in the house." She runs her hand across the surface of the table, pretending to knock off everything in sight. "For a while, Mickey went out to eat. Then eventually he began to eat a little of the stuff, saying, 'Well, I'll have a little of these vegetables' and this and that. I think it probably helped

him an awful lot too, just by osmosis. He's just too lazy to go out all
the time, so it got to where he'd eat whatever junk I made.

"Being a fanatic, like I said—I can't do anything halfway—I went
whole hog. I went around throwing out everybody's canned goods and
saying, 'We're all going to eat Pritikin . . . no more meat, we will not
have any meat in this family.' " To emphasize her point, she raps a
clenched fist purposefully on the table.

The check paid, the three of us leave the restaurant and climb back
into the car. In the front seat, Pam turns around to continue the
conversation. "I wouldn't consider myself fanatically Pritikin now,"
she says, "but I do think I follow a pretty good diet. I'm not fanatical
on anything now. Probably the greatest thing I've learned in all my
life—and it was from the Pritikin Program—is moderation. In everything. Even my food. Before, no matter what you'd put in front of me,
I'd sit and eat it. It didn't matter whether I was hungry. It was just there
and it was gone. And I mean I would be very uncomfortable sometimes
because I had put away too much food." She makes a shallow sound
with her breath as she recalls her old habits.

"Gradually," she begins again, as we settle into her office, "I
learned. In May of 1982, I had the graft put in my arm, and in June, I
had my first dialysis."

Ever a person to create opportunity from adversity, Pam explains
how the dialysis she had to undergo, because of her kidney disease,
helped her monitor her diet. "By that time I was on dialysis on a
regular basis and I found that when I was dialyzed, I could watch my
blood chemistry. They would do chemistry twice a week. I could see in
my lab work what I could eat and what I couldn't, and I'd adjust my
diet that way. I watched the potassiums go up and down, the sodiums,
the choloride levels and I could relate a lot of them to intake of rich
foods like oils, or fats or gravies or that sort of thing. So I really began
to watch, really watch. I'd say to myself, 'OK, I'm going to eat some
meat. I'll be tested tomorrow, let's see what it looks like. Next week,
I'll eat a piece of chicken when I'm going to be tested the following
day, and I know I can see the patterns.' I gradually modified my diet to
sort of get away with a little of each thing, nothing excessive in
anything. I didn't eat too much meat, too much fruit, not too much
starch. If I felt that I wanted something and I would normally have a
serving that was, say, a cup, I would eat half a cup. And I found, as I
did this, that I gradually cut back and felt better. And after I went on
dialysis, my cholesterol level dropped significantly."

As if not to make it sound too perfect, she admits, "I found I was
hungry more often, but that's all right, too. I'll eat a small snack now

and it's so pleasant to feel satisfied but not stuffed and overfull, with your body sluggish for four hours trying to digest a monstrous meal. So with the knowledge from Pritikin and dialysis, I gradually more and more got out of the habit of heavy meals of any kind or an excessive volume of any kind. I cut down and down and down. My normal habit now is I have two meals a day and probably two very light snacks. And I don't eat because it's time to eat anymore. I eat when I'm hungry. I eat when I really feel a necessity."

As she finishes her sentence, two dogs scamper into the room and make a beeline for her purse, where she's stashed some leftovers from breakfast. One dog is a miniature black poodle, the other a mix of odds and ends with short white hair and very quick movements. As she unwraps the snacks, she says, "Momma can't come home without bringing the girls a little treat."

III

"You don't appreciate the various intricacies of the body until it doesn't work."

The mail is all opened and Pam Mulhair has finished stacking it in piles. Across the desk from her, I fiddle with my tapes and wonder what her next task will be. But she sits still now, reaching down occasionally to pet one of the two dogs that sit in the well of the large oak desk. Reviewing the challenges she has faced medically and mindful of her life philosophy, I wonder if she has suffered from depression or fear or anxiety. I ask her if she knows what fear looks like. Her answer has a familiar ring.

"The biggest fear in my life is not being in control of everything," she says, repeating the idea sharply, "not in control." There is a little silence, as we both edge around this thought. Elaborating, she says, "Because there have been very few times in my life when I couldn't control what was happening."

"What," I asked tentatively, "about when the nephrologist told you that you were facing kidney failure?"

"Well," she sighs distantly, "that's something you can't control, but," she adds with more purposeful vigor, "it's also something, as far as I'm concerned, that's not fatal. So it's not out of control because you still have an option. You're not at the point where you have no options left." As if to convince both of us, she starts to tick them off: "You've got transplant, you've got CAPD, you've got hemodialysis." Then she adds a sentence that might well be a warning to anyone flirting with the risks of degenerative disease, "You don't appreciate, I think, the miraculous intricacies of the body until it doesn't work. A kidney doesn't work and you realize how many things this organ called a kidney really did without your ever thinking about it."

She turns and watches some kids come down the street on skate-boards. The dogs are poised to bark as the teenagers come nearer the building. "I find I have a greater awareness and appreciation of these things," she muses gravely, "but I still don't have a fear." Then she grants, speaking rapidly, as if in apology, "Once in a while I have some resentment. I think, 'Why me?' You know. Why? Then I get into something that borders somewhere on a religious belief. I think to myself, 'Why me, when there's all those skid-row bums down there with kidneys that are working 100 percent, and all they're doing is pouring wine into themselves and doing nothing productive. Here I am a productive, active, working, involved human being and I've got to fight this problem too. I've got an additional handicap.' And occasion-ally the thought crosses my mind, 'Hey, you know, this isn't real fair.' " She starts to shift in her chair and I realize that she is holding a bag of urine in her lap and that it is starting to fill up. The heavy plastic bag has been hidden by her sweater up to this point, but I remember that it's now been an hour since we've eaten.

"What do you do with that thought when you get it?" I asked.

"Oh, I don't know," she answers. "I think I look at it, and I say, 'Well, it's not fair, but you've got two choices. You can sit and brood about the fact that it's not fair. Or you can say, 'This is the handicap that I have and was given for whatever reason.' And you pick it up and go on and make the best of it."

And then as if to emphasize her point, she tells the story of her kidney failure. "After I got out of the Pritikin center in September, I went to the Philippines. I had follow-up blood work done when we came back, I think maybe October, and then in December also. Things looked fine. At Christmastime, Mickey and I took the motor home for a couple of weeks and went down to Cabo San Lucas in Baja, Mexico. And I kind of fell off the wagon a little." She hesitates, perhaps struggling to piece together details, or trying to avoid recalling them. "I ate a lot—beans and tacos and good junky Mexican food. And when I got back, I went in for my January blood work. My creatinine levels had gone up to six, just zap, right up the line.

"I never have really been a drinker," she continues. "A heavy week for me would be if I had three or four glasses of wine. In fact there would be months and months where I'd never even have a drink, period. So that had nothing to do with it. But when my GP saw that January blood work, he said, 'You've got to go see a nephrologist, a specialist. Maybe this thing is a fluke again, but I'm inclined to think that's not the case.' And then he said, 'I don't have the expertise to really stay with it now; you need somebody who really knows what they're doing.' "

"What did you think?" I asked.

"Well, I should have been scared," she answered evenly. "But you see, I still didn't buy it. I always thought, 'Well, I guess there's going to be a reprieve. It'll come back.' But they sent me in February to see a nephrologist in Inglewood. He reviewed my medical history and said, 'I am of the opinion that you definitely do have a nephrology problem and it's going to continue to get worse. You should prepare yourself for it. Your choices in life are going to be a kidney transplant, dialysis or CAPD.' " (CAPD is a method of dialysis that uses the peritoneum, the membrane that lines the abdominal cavity and surrounds the stomach, intestines and other digestive organs.)

The room is quiet, cradling the last of her words. You try to think what news like that must mean. Pam confirms her shock. "It kind of hit me then, I think, that maybe I was facing something that wasn't going to be that easily controlled this time or ignored or pushed aside."

She bores on, stonily. "I remember getting rather upset and sort of falling apart in his office, maybe the first or second time we sat and talked. He is very good from the standpoint of taking the time to go through the whole thing, "feeling" out how the patient is responding psychologically and trying to prepare them. He said, 'You need first to prepare yourself mentally for the fact that this is going to happen, and second, you have to make preparation in the event that it happens soon, so that you are ready for it.' What he was talking about was he wanted me to have a graft implanted so that I would have a method of dialysis. Transplants weren't quite as successful back then as they are now because of the new cyclosporine drugs available. So I started with conventional dialysis in a self-care unit where you go in and they train you to use the machinery and everything. You do your own but there's a nurse supervising all the time. Usually someone has to be with you to hook you up."

Mickey pokes his head in and joins the conversation. "I had never stuck a needle in anyone in my life," he says, picking up on Pam's remark about dialysis. "Needles scare me. It turned out it's easy to do. I've never stuck a needle through her vein," he boasts proudly. "I've had problems getting it in but I've always done that. But I care. You don't know whether everyone else is going to care as much as you do. I decided I wanted to buy a machine right then, so we could do it all ourselves."

Pam interrupts him. "I wanted a portable home dialysis unit that we could put in the motor home. But it took a while to get that set up. Then one day when I went in early for my home training in June of '82, they told us about the CAPD system and showed us how it works. I got my portable machine, but I kept thinking about the ease and the simplicity of the CAPD system. And I didn't feel real good on hemo, because it's very hard on your body."

Mickey, following the conversation and continuing to mumble his iconoclastic opinions of doctors and hospitals, adds, "It's a strain too, because you're off a day and on a day."

"Well," explains Pam, "in a matter of a four-hour period, you're pulling all of those toxins out of your body. And you end up feeling washed out and draggy, and it's hard to keep motivated. But the thing that bothered me the most, being as independent as I am, is that I had to depend on somebody else—somebody's tied to you four hours a day, three days a week. And I thought to myself, 'You know it's really not fair to the family, and I don't like it.' So I decided the thing to do would be to have a system that I could handle without any help. It's easier on the body—a more natural method of dialysis because you get constant dialysis action. It's working all the time, twenty-four hours a day, so you don't have peaks and valleys. And it's so simple that it's amazing that it can work."

With CAPD, the peritoneal membrane is used as the filter mechanism of the kidneys. Plastic tubing called a catheter is inserted through the abdominal wall. The dialysis solution is gravity fed into the abdominal cavity and the system is closed off. When it's had time to work—three or four hours—the resulting fluid is gravity-fed out again, bringing out extra potassium and extra calcium and magnesium and phosphorus, the substances that don't belong in the body.

The drawback is that CAPD is an open system into the abdominal cavity and the solution is an ideal growth place for bacteria. "But," Pam says, "I have a procedure that I use to guard against that. I have a bathroom that no one else uses, our little half bath. I sterilize it two or three times a week. I wash it down with bleach or whatever. I have a clean counter top. When I go in, I put my bag that I'm unattaching and my new bag on the counter. I always wear a mask. If there's any question in my mind, if I have to add medications or anything, I disinfect for a minimum of five minutes with Betadine. The spike on the end of the catheter, which is a little grip area with a little prong that actually penetrates the bag, is something you never, never touch under any circumstances because that's where you might induce contamination. When I'm ready to make the transfer, I get the old one ready to actually pull the spike and I pull the sterilized cover off the new one. There's probably not more than a second that that spike is exposed. I started out with good procedure, and I do everything the same way every time, and now it's such a habit I could probably do it in my sleep.''

As Pam describes her precautions, without realizing it you think to yourself, ''Some people could allow this to dominate their life, and here she is describing a complicated and life-supporting procedure like the details of a financial transaction.''

But before dialysis, there was adjustment to the Pritikin life-style. Feeling better and motivated, Pam Mulhair remained on a strict Pritikin diet for half a year after she left the center. Now that her program is modified because of her kidney failure, she says she eats only small meals and drinks little.

''If I eat breakfast, it would be at midmorning,'' she explains. ''A lovely breakfast for me now would be a small piece of fruit, maybe some kind of a veggie, carrot sticks or cauliflower or something crunchy, a nice slice of toast and, some days, cottage cheese. I seem to get real good long-range energy out of that and I find normally that I'm not hungry until maybe two-ish. Then I'll think something sounds good and it will usually be either a piece of orange or a piece of apple or grapefruit, some kind of fruit that kind of fills me up. Maybe if I'm not hungry, or just barely, a couple of soda crackers, something to take the edge off. Because, you see, I get an awful lot of calories—the base of the solution you use for CAPD is dextrose.

''I drink about two cups of coffee a night,'' she continues. ''But for the most part I don't drink a lot of anything anymore. I try to be very careful about my fluids. I do drink apple juice and orange juice. I try to go real light on the orange and grapefruit because of the sugar concentration; it's better for me to actually eat the fruit.

''Dinner is fish, chicken, lots of vegetables, salads. I use lowfat cottage cheese and nonfat milk, sometimes lowfat because Mickey hates the nonfat. We still eat out a lot, and one thing we love is Chinese food—steamed fish and vegetables. We learned that traveling in the Orient.''

She pauses a moment and turns around in her chair to face the window. Then she turns back toward me and addresses herself to a subject to which she has obviously given much thought. "I feel," she starts, "that the biggest salvation America can have is to modify its diet, maybe not as radical as Pritikin, but it really needs to be modified. A good place to start would be to make it mandatory that every restaurant cut its portions by half. People don't need the amount of food they're served. Three times a day and three snacks a day, too. Every time the lunch truck comes through . . . or you're going through a mall, every other store is a fast-food store. And regardless of the exercise craze, most of us do not get the exercise either. We're doing this stuff, stuff, stuff routine."

I wanted to know from Pam, given everything that's happened to her, what her immediate concerns are now.

"Well, this company was my immediate goal," she answers, "building this little company. This one has been a lot of fun because I've managed to look at it at arm's length and therefore it doesn't keep me alive. It's not something that's my child, like the other one was.

"I think I learned a lot from the Pritikin Program about stress," she offers, "because I learned about ways of looking at stress—taking your own stress and setting it out there and looking at it. What is it doing? Why is it doing it? What is pushing my buttons and why? The stress management program was more important to me than any of the rest of the Pritikin Program.

"I always knew I had a problem with stress," she reflects. "But I always just looked at it as me being wound too tight. In fact that's my brother's favorite description when somebody comments on my pace: 'My sister was born with her mainspring wound too tight.' Even as a child, they say I didn't need people to amuse or entertain me. I'd take my nap and when I woke up, I would do productive things like picking all the wallpaper off the wall. I think I took my first trip on my own when I was about three years old. I took my dog and my tricycle and I went to visit my mother's friend two miles away, across a major highway." She laughs and then says, "I kept my mother's heart pumping." Then she pauses again and concludes, "So it was just something about the way my gears were put together.

"At Pritikin," she continues, "working with the psychologist there, I began to see, I think for the first time, that I wasn't the cool, laid-back person I thought I was. I don't ruffle on the surface," she explains. "Now, Mickey, if anything goes wrong, the slightest thing, he blows up all over the ceiling, which is probably better. Consequently maybe he gets it out of his system. Things can go wrong and my tone of voice never changes, my patience level never changes, I just go along very smoothly; I try very calmly to explain things to people.'' Her manner now becomes very calm but patronizing as she imitates herself. '' 'Well, you didn't get it right this time, let's go through it again, because it can be done and we can get it right without any big problems.' I handled all the major problems in my life on that same basis, just calm and collected. That's changed some too. I now allow myself to get irritated; I allow myself to say something to someone when I get irritated at them.

"Part of it was control," she offers, "but I also do not really like blowing up at people. I think I've learned now to be a lot easier on me. That may not be easier on the people around me, and yet in some ways, maybe it is. I think you can be so level sometimes that people don't feel they can react. A lot of that, I think, may have come from my home environment. At only one time in the entire period I was home growing up did I ever hear my mother and father raise their voices at each other. I couldn't have been more than five years old and it stands out like a terrifically vivid memory. They were always so calm.

"I do sort of reach a point in my mind," she says, "where I control and control, and it's very hard for me not to be in control of the situation. I'm very independent, and I imagine I'm certainly not one of the easiest persons in the world to live with, especially if you have any idea of dominating. But I also have a real deep-seated faith. I believe that most of the things that happen, I guess, somehow, God has planned them, in an overall plan that perhaps I don't understand. Perhaps it's beyond my capacity.'' She pauses and then smiles, as if maybe all of this is becoming too heavy. "I do occasionally get into shouting matches with God and I do occasionally ask 'Why?' But I think for the most part this belief is a rock. When something reaches a point that I can't handle or it's out of my control, I can comfortably say, 'I trust you, I believe you, you are my God, you have to be all-knowing, all-seeing, so here, it's yours, take care of it.' I don't know how people survive without this, without whatever they perceive God to be, this entity. That's my Gibraltar, that's my solace, my place that I can run to. I do get frustrated,'' she adds as an afterthought, "when I run into a corner or a brick wall. Like recently my mother's been having some problems.

"She went through a series of difficulties and ended up in a real bad depression. Some of her friends called and told me she was having a lot of confusion and not remembering things and acting really strange. So I talked her into coming down here. She doesn't understand, however, that I still keep a normal schedule and so she went back home. But she wasn't taking care of herself. Eventually I went up and I put her in the hospital and they put her on a program of antidepressant drugs and some sleeping medication because she wasn't sleeping at night.''

There is a quiet period, after which Pam says with a sigh, flicking a paper clip across the desk, ''That was the worst frustration I've had in I can't tell you how long, because it was something I could not control. I couldn't do anything about it. And, you know, no matter how bad I wanted to help her and wanted to try to make her see what was happening, I couldn't do it.''

As I start to ask what kind of a feeling that is, Pam, sitting back in her chair, fakes a mad scream. ''It's like standing and beating your head against the wall. You start chasing yourself. Would it help if I did this? Would it help if I did that?''

Before she can explain any further, the phone rings. She answers it on the second ring. It's a personal call that lasts about ten minutes. As she hangs up the phone, she says, ''I've taken her under my wing, too.'' I observe out loud that she seems to have a lot of people in her life to take care of. ''Yes,'' she answers jovially, ''I'm the godmother of the family.'' I laugh and she responds, ''No, really, if there's a problem, they say, 'Call Godmother Pam.' But I don't mind. It evolved, really. As my mother would say, people gravitate to where they can get their problems solved. If you find the guy whose desk is real clean and neat, you're a little hesitant to put any paper on his desk. But if you see this guy over here with stacks of paperwork . . .'' She cuts herself off, ''So everybody just stacks their paper on my desk.

''It's so automatic for me. There are certain members of the family that I feel responsible for because I want to, because I love them. And because I feel they need the help. There's others I don't worry much about or bother much about because they're capable of doing for themselves or taking care of themselves. This particular lady I was just talking to needs a lot of moral support, a lot of TLC. She's emotionally a little bit fragile, and it's very easy for me to kind of pick her up and dust her off and make sure she's OK and going along fine. She's really a sweetheart, but she just needs a little extra care. She's got some family here, brothers and sisters. But as far as somebody, a child she can kind of hug and hang on to and really feel safe and secure, there isn't anyone. Her daughter is not as warm, I think, and as accessible and as emotional as I am. So she finds this a Linus blanket for her. I'm a security blanket. And if she's down, she tells me, 'I can call you up and talk to you for five minutes and feel great.' ''

She continues, ''I have a nephew who's a genius, literally, probably has a 180 IQ. He was coming home from college in Santa Barbara and had a bad car accident that just laid his head open. He was in a coma for five weeks and we literally had to retrain him to do everything, I mean from brushing his teeth to walking. He was always a little bit skeptical and had a tendency to look down his nose at most people because they couldn't think as quickly as he could and weren't as perceptive. I've often said to him, maybe God had to slow you down a little bit, to show you how to live. I feel a real deep responsibility for him from a protective sense. My sister had three boys and, of course, since she's gone, I'm their mommy.''

"How is it,'' I asked her, "that you never had any children?''

There is a long break in the conversation here. We can hear each other breathing. "I had a little . . .'' she says, then pauses and begins again. "Let's see, I was pregnant in '69, carried her full term and lost her in delivery. Then I found out again in '76 that I was pregnant, and I just couldn't handle it. It had taken me the nine months to psychologically get ready for that first one. I didn't feel that I could do a good job as a career person and a mother so I figured one's got to go, and I talked myself literally into just about handing over my business. I had trained some people, and I decided, 'Well, at least I can go home for the first five years and then maybe, you know, go back to work after the kid is in school.' And it was such a shock psychologically then when I lost her. I had to reverse all this process, go back into thinking, 'Well, now I'm back in the career game.' And I didn't feel I could go through it again in '76. I figured I would be a basket case before my pregnancy was term just worrying about it.''

Against the dense stillness of the office, she continues. "I can only feel it goes back to you've got to have a faith or someplace to hang your troubles or whatever it is. I have to believe that was the way things were supposed to be.'' Her voice drops; she says gently, "Or she would have been fine. One way or the other God had to have a reason. You know, maybe he knows best that I never would have been a good mother, that I would have always hung on to a kid with one hand and tried to hang on to a career with the other. And I'm not sure they always mix well. I think something suffers.'' She adds another, quiet thought, "I don't know, maybe somebody more intelligent than I . . .'' but she doesn't finish.

I left Pam and Mickey Mulhair as I had met them earlier—standing in the hallway of their plant. Mickey had come back in from trouble-shooting some problem or another. He wanted to know if my husband knew anything about dune-buggy racing—his hobby. I told him no. We talked idly a little longer, winding down. Pam leaned against the door of the office. We were standing there, swapping small talk like thousands of other people every day in similar situations. The only difference was that the woman standing in front of me had experienced two heart attacks and kidney failure. And she was talking to me with that open voice, those curious eyes, seemingly oblivious to the fact that in her left arm, wedged against her left hip and attached to her by plastic tubing, she held a full bag of her own urine.

Fatality

There is a calmness about Pam Mulhair not often evident in the majority of men who have had heart attacks. In moments, it almost seems a serenity. Could it be the satisfaction of lessons learned? Certainly she has tested her physical resources to their ultimate. Could illness go much further in dominating her life? And yet you don't feel it. If soul-searching was ever an important element of her coping strategies, it appears to have been replaced by that kind of studied optimism women seem most capable of. Nothing in excess she says now. How could there be, given the complications she has lived with over the years, short though her life has been?

A Type A woman—Type A refined now, as Alan Keiser would say. Pam's story serves as a dramatic warning of the potential dangers of a pace we have mindlessly established in our contemporary life. Her bad diet led to diabetes, which led to the small vessel disease that affected her kidneys. The high cholesterol that often accompanies diabetes affected her blood pressure and contributed to the development of the atherosclerosis that caused her heart atacks. Cigarettes, little exercise, high cholesterol. Diabetes, high blood pressure, kidney failure. Around and around—a lethally dangerous game to play, where ironically the control so desired by Type A men—and women—is lost in a muddle of confusing illness.

"I don't walk on a regular basis now," Pam says, "even though I know I should. Because there's the blood loss problem. But I do get a lot more exercise than I did. A lot more, even though it's mostly limited walking. I do some bicycling, but I find walking is probably better for me. It's not as strenuous; it's kind of a nice rhythm and I can amble along and adjust, according to where my blood level happens to be at the time, as far as maintaining a brisk pace or not as brisk. And I don't eat like I did before Pritikin," she adds softly.

Mickey, who is obviously an important factor in the Mulhair equation, says, "We like Chinese food, fish . . ."

"Steamed fish," Pam clarifies. "And Chinese vegetables. With traveling to the Orient, I've also gotten used to a basic Chinese diet. There it's very easy to get and I like it a lot. You've got all these nice vegetables. I really like vegetables and now I find that I recently got on a real bad fruit kick. Grapefruit and oranges."

"Yeah," Mickey complains, "I started eating grapefruit because she'd eat the whole damn thing. Like last night, she cut the grapefruit and asked me, 'Do you want half of this?'—like 'You'd better not want half of this.' So I said, 'Yeah, I'll take it.' "

Mickey worries about Pam's medication. "If you take a lot of pills," he says, "it seem like it creates a lot of problems. Pam takes a lot of pills. She takes all kinds of pills, but she has to take them." He dryly adds another one of his iconoclastic medical opinions, "I'm assuming she does because some genius told her she had to."

Pam laughs. "About ninety percent of the time," she says, "he's not sure what the hell's going on."

But Mickey's not giving up. "In the evening she takes a pill to . . ."

"But she's still up and around," I venture.

"Oh yeah, she's moving," Mickey says. "She has kidney failure but how did it come on? None of her family has kidney failure. I imagine that's connected with diabetes."

Pam corrects him. "No, I have serious kidney problems in my family. Besides what Carl had, Gertie also had bad kidney problems."

Undaunted, Mickey asks, "Are Gertie's kidneys still there?"

"Gertie's not still here," Pam answers.

Pam Mulhair died on September 30, 1985. She was at home with Mickey when she experienced her third and fatal heart attack. The nitroglycerin she took for her angina was not sufficient this time. Time— the enemy of the heart attack victim. Within an hour of her first symptoms, Pam was dead—no time for the paramedics who had helped her before. No time for the emergency room.

There can be no doubt that Pam Mulhair was a special person. She had a love and zest for life that refused to be daunted by a complex of illnesses that would have thwarted a lesser person. To the end, she refused to believe that sheer force of her powerful will could not keep her going. Dr. Anderson, her GP and friend over the years, acknowledges Pam's belief that she could win the battle with the small vessel disease that was the source of her problems. "She had this idea always that she was going to beat the disease," he remembers. "My dream for her was that she would eventually be well enough to have a heart and kidney transplant. Pam's vision was that she could live it out experiencing a series of only small attacks, watching herself.

"She was becoming *very* incapacitated," he continues, "before she went to the Pritikin center; and as busy as she was, she felt she had to go in. She greatly improved her activities after the Pritikin Program; she did things she could never have done before she went to the center. Her quality of life improved considerably. I have never encountered such an individual as she was—always going to conquer a new horizon. The average person would have died two years before, or even before she went into the center. Her life was probably prolonged by the things she learned at the center and the things that she did afterwards. She was constantly aware of her cholesterol and triglycerides."

The Pam Mulhair I know is not dead. Her spirit lives on in these pages, in her indomitable belief in her own power to survive. I believed her when she spoke of her determination to beat the illness that beset her, even though I knew full well the seriousness of her afflictions. I still see Pam as I did that last day, in those gray slacks and that baggy red sweater, her eyes sparkling. Strong, sensitive, giving. "She was like a sister to everyone," says Dr. Anderson. Intelligent, resolute and full of life, despite her sick body's attempts to cheat her out of it.

Today she rests in the soil of Oregon. What luck that her words live on to inspire others. She would have cared about each and every one of you.

Chapter 6

Martin Stone, 56, chairman of Adirondack Corporation and World Paper, Inc., Chief Executive Officer, Monogram Industries, 1961–83. Married, two children.

Diagnosis: hypercholesterolemia

I

"I was virtually certain that I would have a heart attack by fifty."

Statistics corroborate the fear. Each year, well over a million people in this country are stricken by a heart attack. For many it will be the first attack, the warning. For others it will be fatal. Every year as many as 550,000 Americans die from this dreaded affliction. Almost 50 million Americans have some form of heart or blood vessel disorder. Before cancer even, heart disease remains our number one killer. HEART DISEASE: identified by the World Health Organization as "the greatest epidemic mankind has faced."

The individuals whose stories have been presented here are familiar with the effects of this malady. Alan Keiser almost lost his life; Jim Irwin his desire to live. Jack Rutta changed his life to avoid its effects. Fred Rizk still wrestles with the monkey on his back. Pam Mulhair remained alive and kicking, it seems, by sheer force of her own will. The experiences of these brave individuals offer inspiration and hope. The final member of this diverse crew, however, the final actor in this play of passion and courage, tells a tale of woefully different proportions, his circumstances fundamentally different in their scope and ramifications.

Martin Stone fought, not against the infirmity the others courted and then fought; he struggled not with the demon of incapacity nor the fiend of troubling self-awareness, nor the frustration of attempting to avoid further suffering. His is a saga of totally different proportions. It is the story of the fear of heart disease and of one man's well-meaning but misdirected efforts to address this fear head on—a tale of good intentions gone peculiarly astray.

It has been said that the fear of heart disease has approached the level of a phobia in contemporary society, second in its persuasiveness only to our fear of cancer. Four years ago, however, according to the National Center for Health Statistics, 989,610 deaths were attributable to heart disease. Cancer claimed less than half that number—422,720 people in the same year. Fear, however, does not necessarily translate into motivation for action. Commitment to act involves decision-making, which further requires acknowledgment of a problem and its potential effects. As we have seen with people like Pam Mulhair and Alan Kesier, denial is a seductive strategy. Denial, at its core, depends on emotional reaction; it is void of the security of the calculated risk. Denial is a strategy so all-pervasive that even if the feared event comes to pass—the heart attack, the recurrent angina—denial continues to exert its fearful influence.

Denial's opposite is awareness, the calculated percentage, the prudent choice. Related to heart disease, it suggests reduction of risk factors, enhancing chances for good health. But such insurance does not come cheap. Its price tag includes acknowledging limits, recognizing diminishing options. Most of all, it involves vulnerability—to the realities of one's personal responsibility. Listen to one person who opted for awareness over denial. Listen to how one individual's informed consciousness sadly becomes an obsession. Understand how well-intentioned, practical strategies to avoid heart disease influenced Martin Stone and his family, to the point that Connie Stone, his wife, says, "He began to calculate all decisions based on how long he would live."

Martin Stone's story lacks the overt drama of the Keisers' life-and-death struggle or Pam Mulhair's tight determination to hold on to life. His story has a cold, steel edge to it. It is not the stuff of emotions, of carelessly made decisions, of lost hope. Rather, it is an account of a fiercely disciplined, intellectual determination in the service of the goal of avoiding heart disease. The element of fear lies buried under a gains-and-loss approach to avoiding the inevitable, for it was Stone's belief, based on his family history, that he would have a heart attack by age fifty and would probably be dead by midlife. This was not idle speculation, but a well-considered opinion based on assessment of the evidence, undertaken by an extremely intelligent, informed individual.

For better or worse, most of us see life as infinite, stretching before us with endless opportunities. Only as midlife approaches do thoughts of our mortality invade our thinking. Imagine, however, how it would be to travel down life's road with prescribed limits on your journey from the very start, the signposts marked, anticipation thwarted. To temper dreams of your personal goals with the sure realization that you will only travel so far; that you will never see your children grown, for example. Imagine that your obsession is so great that you may not recognize its effects on others around you. If you can do that, you can imagine what life was like for Martin Stone.

Fortunately the precautions Stone implemented against the inevitable appear to have averted his personal catastrophe. But this is only part of the story. As in each of these dramas, we must reckon with the supporting cast. And as always, the second level of players was far from immune to suffering. For a young wife—anticipating a loving family, shared companionship, exciting challenges—the future should have been rosy. Not so. For years, Connie Stone endured her husband's fixation, sharing only its downside—the constant fear of imminent death or diminished capacity. Her life was overshadowed with this fearful inevitability, based on two seemingly rock-solid factors: Stone's family history of heart disease and his own high cholesterol. Connie lived with her husband's misgivings, afraid to evaluate the possibility of the inevitable and yet without any physical evidence to bolster his calculated predictions.

Martin Stone's heart disease never manifested itself further than heredity and history—no heart attack lent credence to his apprehensions; no failed stress test, no angina, no questionable electrocardiogram. Only his obsession.

If the Stones appear dispasssionate in their story, it is partly their style of dealing with life. Reason prevails in the Stone household, sensible logic that appears to engender a particularly comfortable form of security. Their apparent nonchalance would also seem to be related to the inevitable weight of living all those years under this burdensome pressure. Unlike the Keisers, whose past struggles have created an acute definition of the present, the implications of the Stones' story are more oblique. One might be tempted to suggest that it would be better buried, locked in an airtight vault and forgotten. For the Stones themselves, perhaps this might appear a comfortable strategy. For others, however, their story unfolds here as yet further evidence of the powerful grip that heart disease, the twentieth century epidemic, continues to tighten around contemporary Western society.

"Once I was almost killed in a river boat accident," Stone explains as he begins to tell his story, "and it was the most extraordinary experience imaginable. A betting man would have had to say that my chances of survival were one in a hundred in that situation. And I don't know how but we made it.'' He hesitates a moment and then continues to recount the drama of his experience.

"It was like I was on drugs," he says, "because everything was terribly vivid. The flowers were redder and more yellow and more orange. The grass was greener. I hugged everybody. I loved life and I loved everybody. Standing on a rock waiting for rescue, I spent the whole night dancing. It was being unbelievably happy at being alive. And I watched as the year went by, and that sensitivity to life declined to the point that although I could see that I still would never be quite the same, it wasn't like the weeks immediately after it happened. And in a way, I was very unhappy that it had declined, because it was a wonderful experience. And so I know damn well that when I expected life to be relatively short for me, till age fifty or fifty-two or fifty-five, I think I valued life more highly than I otherwise would have and lived it more fully. So I think there are advantages as well as disadvantages to that.''

Although this heightened sense of life's value may have enriched Martin Stone's perception—a result of his prediction of an early death—such insight was not necessarily extended to his wife. "I don't know," Connie says, "what it was like for Marty personally during that time, but going through that for me . . .'' She melts back into her chair and looks forlorn. "We had everything in the world to live for. We loved each other a lot and had a wonderful, extraordinary life. But it was like living with a hammer over your head. Living with a feeling in the pit of your stomach all the time that the other shoe was going to drop, that things were too perfect, too nice.'' She adds lifelessly, "I mean, there was this big black cloud that hung over our heads all the time.

"That," she continues to reflect, "was maybe the most difficult part of life with him. I was just living in terror all the time. When I was pregnant with Sam, our first child, he was so convinced—no one was ever more convinced—that he was going to have a heart attack at some point in his life, very early.''

Her husband interrupts her. "I figured," he says, "before fifty or by fifty.''

"When I was pregnant with Sam," Connie continues, "at the beginning of the pregnancy, Marty would say things like, 'Well, if I don't see him . . .' And then when I was eight-and-a-half months pregnant, a particularly vulnerable time, one night he came in and sat down and told me, 'I think I'm having a heart attack.' We had to rush him to the hospital.''

Stone justifies himself: "I had all the symptoms." Connie looks slightly exasperated, but allows him to explain. "It turned out that somehow or another, with all the extreme exercise I was doing, I had bruised some sensitive areas in my chest. And when I breathed to the absolute maximum, when I expanded my lungs, they rubbed against this one area and it gave the exact same symptoms of a heart attack." Sitting across from him, Connie listens quietly to his description. "The hospital people thought I was having a heart attack," he continues, "but none of the EKGs or anything showed it. The thing was that I was having gigantic pains—crushing pains—here," he says as he points to his chest, "and pains down the left arm."

"This," remembers Connie, "was two weeks before I had our son."

Listening to Martin Stone's words, I reflected speculatively that although most people drawn to the Pritikin Program have been activated by the incentive of actual serious illness, that doesn't appear to apply in his case.

But he stops me tersely. "I was seriously ill from a mental standpoint," he says. "You see, I was mentally ill and mentally off balance." His wife looks at him suspiciously, as if she has never heard this before. "I'm glad this is on tape," she ventures as her husband continues. "No," he insists, "those kind of people have an extraordinary strong compulsion about having been seriously ill that made them willing to accept the discipline of this diet. Well, I had lived with the mental anguish of this thing hanging over my head for all these years. I had my father's experience that weighed so heavily, and therefore I was willing to put up with the privations of all of this, which I don't even regard as privations."

His forthright revelations strike me as an incredible proposition. I asked Connie what all of this did to her.

"I was angry, really angry for a long time about it," she responds. "I would tell him, 'We can't live this way, I can't live with somebody who leads the healthiest life of anyone you've ever seen and who is convinced that he's going to keel over any moment.' "

When I asked if there were any way to solve it, Connie says, "Not that I knew, none."

"You had no symptoms?" I asked her husband.

"No," he answers.

"No angina or anything like that?" I persisted.

"No," he repeats. "But as I said, one thing it did was give me an appreciation for time that was important and it also made life much more vivid."

* * *

To reach Martin and Connie Stone, I flew cross-country to Boston, took a puddle-jumping commuter airline to Burlington, Vermont, rented a dented car, crossed Lake Champlain on a sky-scraping bridge and drove two hours over mountain roads, arriving finally at Last Chance Ranch Road outside Lake Placid, New York.

Passing under the peculiarly Western crossbar that identified the ranch, I drove what seemed another mile or so through rolling meadows, ringed on all sides by pine trees, to a small complex of buildings. By this time, I had crossed a small stream, passed some grazing beef cattle and attempted to feel at home under a menacing Adirondack sky.

I had grown up vacationing in the Adirondack Mountains so the old rough-log lodge buildings were familiar. This vast amount of cleared land, however, was to me an Adirondack anomaly—so much meadow in an area that is usually heavily forested. Martin Stone owns 1,000 acres of this beautiful country, and on it he raises thoroughbred horses. It seems a strange place for a born-and-bred Californian to call home, but as I was soon to learn, nothing is simple with Martin Stone.

There were no signs. The road in front of me headed uphill and vanished among more cleared land and pines. I decided to take a chance on what was immediately in front of me. I turned left off the main road and started up a gravel-covered driveway. There were a number of buildings, some more easily distinguished as to their purpose—what looked like barns, cabins, an office. Stone, I knew, was waiting for me in one of them. Which one was the trick. I passed one or two and decided to turn around and try a building to my left that looked the most like an office. As I turned the car around, I could see a screen door open. A large dog flopped out, followed by a middle-aged man in a blue velour jogging suit. I completed my turn-around and edged the car into the spot my host was gesturing at. We shook hands. He pointed out the dent in my rental car. "What happened?" he asked. "Did you have an accident?"

"No," I answered, wondering at first what he was talking about. We both inspected the car. "Be careful they don't charge you for it," he advised. I agreed to take care, embarrassed to admit that I hadn't checked the car before I drove it away from the small parking lot at the Burlington airport. I followed him back into his office where we both sat down and exchanged pleasantries. Stone sat behind a big desk in a room that fulfilled all my fantasies about the old Adirondack lodges— rough interior, defined spaces. "We're going up the hill for lunch," he explained. Then with no choice offered, he said, "We'll take your car," providing no explanation of what was uphill, or who or what might be waiting for us. Just up the hill; so we went.

At the end of another mile or so of winding road we found the Stone family residence, set in among more evergreens and hardwoods; some spring flowers blossomed and relieved the wildness. From the outside, the house looks like the other buildings, with the rough exterior of a log cabin. Inside, it is warm and inviting. The focal point of the huge kitchen into which we stepped is a large skylight. The room needs it, I thought, for days when the sun steadfastly refuses to appear. It would be dark in here on days like this, even given the light woods with which the interior is finished. A young woman with long dark hair was at work at one of the counters lining the periphery of the room.

So, up the hill meant lunch in the Stone country kitchen, among well-polished silver and antique furniture. It's a cozy place populated with a display of the latest culinary gadgets, including blenders and choppers and a pasta-making machine. Stone makes no introductions but signals his wife to ascend from the basement and join us for lunch. Up she comes after he gives the light switch a few quick flicks. I washed my hands and combed my hair in a small bathroom off the kitchen, smoothed out my clothes and followed the Stones to the table.

After some brief small talk, we delve quickly into the subject of my visit.

"I went to the Santa Monica Pritikin Center for the first time in about 1978," Stone recalls. "I had always had very high cholesterol—in the 275–290 range. And my father's family had been plagued with not only high cholesterol but a lot of heart disease at relatively young ages. My grandmother on my father's side died of a heart attack. And my father had a massive coronary at forty-three. He died on the operating table many years later from heart failure. By then he was sixty-eight."

Sitting in his handsome kitchen, with the mellow Adirondack light seeping through the windows, Martin Stone hardly looks like an obsessive individual. On the contrary, he exudes the air of being altogether comfortable with himself. To judge by his surroundings, things are well managed around him—no helter-skelter environment this. Objects, both practical and decorative, are in their place. A kind of personalized good taste fills the room, adding a different dimension to the aloofness that was my first impression. But his reputation precedes him. I know life was not always this way.

Connie Stone is almost fifteen years younger than her husband. A petite blonde with short wavy hair, she shines with the wholesomeness of the Midwest. Today she is dressed in blue jeans and a long-sleeved T-shirt proclaiming the virtues of the University of Southern California. She exudes a naturalness that at once induces me to feel at home, despite the 3,000 miles that separate me from Los Angeles.

The first course arrives. Pea soup. Between spoonfuls, Stone confirms that he has never had angina. In fact, except for high cholesterol, he has never had any indication of heart disease.

"But," he begins, "I am firmly convinced to this day, that based on all the statistical studies I've read, the Cleveland Clinic studies and all the others . . ." He cuts himself off and starts again. "I had talked to Bill Castelli who runs the Framingham study," he says and then returns to his original idea. "The Cleveland Clinic studies indicated that if you take a computerized run on a male who's fifty and who's had a cholesterol of beween 250 and 300 for twenty-five or thirty years, the chances are like eighty-five percent of his having a heart attack before fifty-two." He pauses to let that thought sink in, completing the idea with its personal ramifications for himself. "And I was certain, with my high cholesterol, that was going to happen to me. There isn't a male member of my father's family who did not have a heart attack before age fifty."

It could be said that modern medical science has initiated great strides in the area of predicting heart disease. Although exact correlations are difficult to establish, epidemiological studies such as the thirty-five-year-old Framingham study, which has monitored 5,209 participants thirty to sixty-five years old—and all healthy when the study began—have documented the relationship between suggested risk factors and heart disease. The Framingham study has determined that generally the higher the blood cholesterol the greater the risk of heart disease, finding, for example, that residents of this small New England town with a blood cholesterol of 230 are twice as likely to suffer from eventual heart disease as those whose cholesterol is 180. Over 300, the risk is four times greater. Interestingly, however, a related study, sometimes referred to as "Son of Framingham," has thus far suggested that environment is more important than heredity for most cardiovascular risk factors.

On the other hand, evidence from other sources suggests that a heart attack suffered by a parent while that individual was still in his forties generally indicates a predisposition to heart disease in his son or daughter. The data also suggest that a man who has a family history of heart disease and who is living a sedentary life runs a fifty percent or better risk of developing heart disease.

While listening to the Stones, and speculating on Martin Stone's predictions for himself, I wondered how the two of them met and happened to settle in Lake Placid.

Stone takes a disinterested stab at the date. "It was in 1970, something like that."

Connie knows precisely. "We met in 1970. And we started living together thirteen years ago." It's a straight answer, no elaboration, so I pursued the question of how and when they decided to slow down the pace of their life and move to Last Chance Ranch.

"Well," he answers slowly, "I think I just got to a point where I felt that I was not going to live very much longer." It's a dramatic and provocative statement from an individual who appears to be so self-contained. But Stone seems deadly serious. I'm prepared to wait for him to finish the thought before evaluating it, but Connie Stone steps in, ready to steal a few lines. "He started judging things that way," she says, "making decisions about what he—we—were going to do." She continues, "He was constantly asking himself, 'Should I do this or that if I have only six more months to live? Is that how I want to live it?' "

"That's right," her husband confirms, reaching for a whole-wheat roll, the shape and configuration I recognize from the Santa Monica Pritikin Center. "I was going to run for governor of California. I campaigned for four months for the nomination, and I think I could have won it. But I thought to myself, 'I hate this.' " The words are charged with genuine feeling. "And I said, 'If I have only four or eight more years to live, do I want to live those four or eight years as governor of California?' " He answers his own question. "I said, 'Hell, no.' Then I asked myself, 'I may only have four or eight more years to live, so what am I doing?' " The detachment with which he approaches this idea is predictable; no mention is made of being fearful of death, only the desire to spend his allotted time well. It's obvious that Martin Stone is a man who knows the word control.

I asked Stone what life was like living that way.

"I don't know," he answers. "I had just lived with it for so long that I didn't . . ."

But Connie is more direct. "He just accepted it," she discloses. "That was what was the worst thing. He was incredibly fatalistic about it. I mean, it was just an accepted fact. It was like everything else; he would try to explain it to me logically." She adds after a pause, "And he can be very logical."

When I wonder what it's like to live with someone who thinks like that, her response is quick and precise. "It was torture," she says. "I mean it was absolute torture. At first, I would go off by myself and cry. I would say to him, 'Don't speak to me that way.' But he would try to make me go over our financial situation so that I'd understand it, and I would say, 'Leave me alone; I can't deal with this.' And then he would say to me, 'You're not being realistic.' "

Asked if this is similar to a cancer patient being informed that he or she has only so many years to live, Connie turns quickly toward her husband. "Do you think there's any difference?" she asks him.

"I don't know," he responds. "In my situation, at least I could still be vigorous. I was not sick." He thinks it through a bit further. "I guess it could be like that," he says, pausing again and then revealing, with some compassion, "You've got to realize that from the time I was eighteen, I expected my father to die anytime. I was with him all the time; I was going through his heart disease with him."

Connie interrupts. This is obviously a well-discussed scenario between them. "He said he was afraid to make his father angry because if he became angry, he might have a heart attack." She hesitates a moment and then adds, with a wink in her voice, "I'm sure it never affected me that way, Marty."

Martin Stone is a pleasant-looking man, with fine salt and pepper gray hair and a compact body. There is a slight touch of a hunch in his posture, or perhaps it is a symptom of years of perpetual forward motion. Obviously he's in good shape. Sitting across from us at the head of the dining table in his comfortable kitchen, he recites his family history casually, almost as if it has little bearing on him. The table is set in front of a large stone fireplace, in a dining area that is separated from the working part of the kitchen, where the dark-haired woman—who turns out to be Mary, the Stones' cook—is industriously at work.

"After his attack," Stone continues, "my father read everything he could on the subject of heart disease. He came to the same conclusion as Nathan Pritikin—that the real problem was diet, specifically fat in the diet, and cholesterol. He also reasoned that the heart was a muscle and that any muscle left unexercised would atrophy. He concluded that the best way to strengthen a muscle was through use, through exercise. He had only half a heart muscle left after his coronary, and he felt that he had to set up a strenuous exercise program. He started with walking. At first, I used to accompany him on the walks. We would walk a block and sit down on the curb and rest. That was as far as he could walk. This was about 1946 . . . so I guess I was eighteen at the time."

Connie listens to the conversation while she makes her way through her large bowl of pea soup. "I remember," she says in her small voice, diminished further by a bout with laryngitis, "Marty used to tell me how terrified he was that his father was going to have a heart attack while they were walking around. He used to tell me about being really scared at that age to take him on a walk."

Offering no comment on his wife's remarks, Stone continues with his commentary. This appears to be a common pattern between them. Unlike Bea and Alan Keiser, where Bea provides the narration and Alan the humorous relief, Stone leads the discussion, and his wife fills in details, referring many of her remarks back to him in a personal way, almost as if he might evaluate the thought before she sets it free. This implies a kind of subtle intimacy between them that otherwise might not be obvious.

Her husband continues, finished with his soup before either of us. "But eventually he got up to walking about eight to ten miles a day," he says. "It took him about six months. He worked as a registered nurse at Columbia Pictures, and he would walk to the studio and walk back. The studio was on Gower in Hollywood, and I used to walk there with him and keep him company. Or my mother would drop me off at the studio and my brother and I would walk home with him. There was just the four of us, my mother and father and my younger brother and I.

"Then after my father retired, my mother and he would get up at five o'clock every morning and walk vigorously and fast—four miles an hour for ten miles, two-and-a-half hours. In addition to the ten miles a day, he would do fifty push-ups and fifty sit-ups a day. He was in extraordinary physical condition. He also put himself on a very low cholesterol diet."

From Stone's description, the habits of the father have been transferred to the son, a man also motivated by the serious pursuit of weighty subjects. "But in the last years," he continues, "his arteries started closing up and I suggested he have bypass surgery. He felt, however, that he didn't have any open arteries left in his body. Now, I don't know how he knew that, but he said he could tell by the way it felt in his legs—he had pains in the legs walking. He told me two weeks before he died that the end was near. We were taking a walk and he was telling me that he was having pains now in his legs and was even starting to have pain in his chest. I think he expected to die at that point."

I asked if his father had discussed his program with his doctors.

"He did," Stone answers, "but they all gave him advice he didn't like, so he rejected it." It appears that independence of thought is also a Stone family legacy. "When he first had the heart attack in 1946, the only place he could afford to go was the veterans' hospital. He was a Navy vet. The doctors there told my mother that he had at most a year to live. And that he had to live a very sedentary life. But he was unwilling to do that and said he didn't think it was even wise. His reasoning was that having half a heart muscle he had better strengthen what he had. The doctors, of course, were telling him just the opposite.

"He explained all of this to me," Stone continues eagerly. "We used to read together. We read all the medical books about cholesterol and all the scientific studies on animals. I used to go to the library and get him books. I was interested," he goes on, breaking apart another whole-wheat roll. "He thought it was going to affect me too. He said, 'I think it affects all of us in this family.'

"And I believed that. I always ate fairly moderately. Up until that point I'd eaten the normal junk, but from then I was fairly careful. You have to remember that was 1946. I've been relatively careful with my diet for thirty-nine years but I've still always had high cholesterol. In fact, I have a mild form of a condition that the doctors describe as hypercholesterolemia. Even a very modest amount of fat or cholesterol causes my serum cholesterol to rise."

Mary clears the soup bowls and replaces each with a dinner plate on which she has arranged our entree—salmon loaf with mushroom sauce. There is also steamed cauliflower on the plate and Jim Irwin's least favorite vegetable, steamed carrots. It looks appetizing. I take a moment to appreciate it. Stone digs in.

Two years earlier, in a telephone conversation, Marty Stone had told me that he was contemplating selling off some of his holdings and planning to move to Lake Placid. He was then living in Massachusetts, in a Boston suburb, and commuting routinely to Los Angeles. Compared to the congestion of L.A., suburban Boston sounded like a fine idea, but having invested in the Adirondack property as a summer home, the Stones fell in love with the area and decided to move there permanently. Although he didn't say so explicitly in that conversation, Stone implied that the Adirondack move was another in his continuing personal ambition to reduce his work involvement and pressure.

Given the Stones' motivation for their move to the ranch, I expected a correlation with its name. Last Chance Ranch, however, had been christened long before the Stones bought it by a rancher who settled in the Adirondacks from the town of Last Chance Gulch, Montana. Last Chance, now bearing the more discrete name of Helena, was the last stand of a group of miners panning for gold. Fatefully, they found the gold they sought and the town of Last Chance thrived. The Montana rancher who brought the town's name to this lush valley in New York State's mountains selected the site because it reminded him of the the West, hence the uncharacteristic crossbar I had noticed when I entered the ranch and the large amount of cleared land. As Stone explained this to me, I remembered that the ranch barns were similar to those I had seen in Western states and that the log buildings I noticed on the property were actually more reminiscent of low-ceilinged Western cabins than the two-story buildings that typically characterize Adirondack "camps."

I asked Martin Stone what his life was like before they moved to the ranch and whether stress had been included in his mortality calculations.

"Yes," he maintains, "I calculated stress, too. Until about 1975 or '76 my life was extraordinarily stressful." (Stone has a way of enunciating multisyllabic words so that syllables receive equal notice, so extraordinary comes out extra-ordinary.) "I was running a conglomerate company with about twenty-nine separate operating divisions and going through a divorce. I led a very, very stressful, demanding life. I traveled an enormous lot. I was a workaholic until about 1972 or '73, and then I started cutting way back."

Pressed, Stone maintains that when he was in the heyday of his activities, he didn't feel particularly stressed. "Not terribly, no," he says complacently. Then he admits, "Times I did; there were rare times when I did."

Connie offers a contrary opinion. "Looking at it from somebody else's perspective," she volunteers, "I don't think people would have believed that you didn't feel stressed, because you were going at such a pace. Other people just don't do that." This is the first of a number of routine statements that Connie will make in which she refers to outside criteria and opinions as a yardstick for her and her husband's opinions of his behavior.

I ask Martin and Connie if they could describe a typical day during the high-stress, Los Angeles period.

"Oh," he begins, as if his schedule was not particularly noteworthy, "I usually ran to the office. It was four miles from home to the office. Then I took a shower, after offending everybody in the elevator on the way up."

Connie laughs, remembering the complaints.

"As a matter of fact," says her husband, "when they built our new office building in Santa Monica and we were going to move over to it, they specifically told me they would not allow running clothes in the elevator." Connie adds, speaking to her husband, "You had a secretary who quit on her second day because you smelled so bad when you came in."

Stone continues. "They were going to provide me with a shower and a changing room in the basement, so I could go up in a fitting fashion in the elevator." Like Jim Irwin, Martin Stone has a way of pushing the conversation forward with summarizing statements. He issues one now, dismissing the shower incident in order to continue his

description. "But anyway, I would run to work and then I would go just
flat out until about twelve-thirty. I suppose from eight-thirty to twelve-
thirty I would handle about five calls an hour at least, so that would be
twenty or more phone calls in that time. Then I would have at least one
person an hour that I met with . . ." Across from me, Connie shakes
her head no.

"More?" he asks.

"Yes," she says.

He seems to accept her correction and continues. "The executives
would come in and I would discuss things with them. I would have
meetings all day, and in between all of this, I would be taking all my
phone calls and dictating. Lunch was always a business lunch. In the
afternoon there would be a meeting every hour and at the same time I
would have those constant phone calls. And then probably at about six
or seven in the evening, I would run home."

"We didn't have any children then," says Connie. "But in the
evening there was always an Urban Coalition or a Common Cause
meeting or something to do besides his reading." She turns to address
her husband in that peculiar way she has of referring the conversation
back to him. "You never stopped until eleven-thirty or twelve."

He agrees. "There was always a lot of reading. And I always
slept six or seven hours a night. I fall asleep instantaneously, anywhere
I want to."

As her husband finishes describing his schedule, Connie enlightens
the past with the present. "He still reverts sometimes. There'll be
periods . . ." She lets that fall and begins again with a positive. "He's
real aware of it now. I really think that is due, too, to the stress
management lectures and the reading he's done, but the thing that
started it was Pritikin. It started with his terrible fear of a heart attack.
He's so logical that he could say, 'This is something I must change if
I'm going to logically attack the problem of not wanting to die by the
time I'm fifty.' More than anybody I know he has the capability to think
that way. But when we were first together, he was driven, I mean really
driven.

"It was hard for me, real hard," she remembers with a sigh. "I
just can't live like that. Our relationship now isn't like that. But I can
remember, especially in the beginning, a song came out by Kris
Kristofferson and Rita Coolidge that said something like, 'You've got to
make time for love.' I remember one time just crying and saying to
him, 'We can't live like this.' I only had ten minutes to get ready to go
over to Max Factor's house for dinner. All day we'd been in meetings
together, and I figured out for the next two weeks we weren't going to

see each other alone. I can remember telling him, 'Listen to this song and listen to what I'm trying to tell you, and please . . .' "

I ask how long it took for him to hear.

"Years," she answers blandly, but with the positive satisfaction that eventually her fears were acknowledged.

I wondered if, given his pace and his history, Connie ever feared that her husband might indeed have a heart attack. "Oh," she answers instantly, "he made me believe it. He's the most convincing man when he wants to be." She turns from me to her husband and says, "But I think the change in you, gradually, from your stress and the pace you lived over the past years is really remarkable; I don't know any of your friends that have done that."

Although he maintained a tight and stressful business schedule, Martin Stone was not without opportunities for recreation. A fanatic baseball fan and well known in Los Angeles, he discloses, "I used to go to sports events on occasion. Some days when the Dodgers were in town, I'd go to Dodger Stadium at around four-thirty, get out on the field at five and pitch batting practice and work out till about seven. Then I'd take a shower and go home. I'd do the running and the stretching and all that. On those days I wouldn't run in the morning." He thinks a minute, reflecting. "I pitched batting practice for the Dodgers about three days a week when they were home. And then when we moved to Boston, I would do the same thing for the Red Sox. And every Sunday I would play baseball."

I asked where the urge for such hectic activity originated.

He doesn't hesitate, his answer a kind of universal banner for his generation. "It comes from the Depression," he volunteers easily. "My father's business went bankrupt and we didn't have any money. And although I never understood life as being particularly difficult—somehow or another we always had enough to eat—for me life was wonderful because I always had a bunch of kids to play with and stuff like that. But for my parents it was very difficult and my father used to tell me stories about how tough things were in the Depression and that nobody had a job. I guess it rang a bell. Also, from the time I was a kid, I had to work because I had to provide a certain amount of income for the family."

Stone leans against the back of his chair, a dining room chair with arms; having finished his meal, he pushes himself away from the table. He crosses his legs, settles his hands in his lap, folded, and thinks a minute. "I did everything," he says. "I had a paper route and I did gardens and then I worked at a carpet factory cleaning the factory. You know, just the kind of things kids do. But,'' he adds with some satisfaction, "I always had a job from the time I was about eight or nine years old, and it always had to be a productive job, because the family always needed money. It had to be a money-producing job.'' Before I can ask another question, he interjects one of his summarizing statements. "So, like a lot of other people from that generation—kids that grew up then—you had stamped on you this desperate desire to create financial security.''

Connie had been listening to the conversation and corroborating her husband's remarks with short nods of her head and a few meaningful glances my way. I suspect that one element in Stone's eventual decision to slow down his pace might be attributed to his relationship with his wife, although if this is true it may have long ago become camouflaged among other issues.

Marty Stone was born and grew up in Los Angeles, which he describes as "until 1955 . . . the prettiest spot on earth. You had clear skies, you had ski mountains right nearby, you had the ocean, the desert. Incredible weather.'' He went to UCLA as an undergraduate, did graduate work at the University of Southern California and graduated from Loyola Law School. In 1961 he joined Monogram Industries, where he worked until he took over the company in 1971. He began as legal counsel and gradually moved over to business management. Stone remembers that he took the company from $5 million to $200 million a year, from 200 to 5,000 employees. He sold his interest in 1983 to go on to other ventures. In the late seventies, he established *California Business* magazine to fill what he characterizes as a need for a publication covering small and medium-sized businesses.

"I have always had this thing about organizing other people's activities,'' he says amiably. "For example, we didn't have Little League when I was a kid and I loved to play baseball. So I organized a baseball team and we practiced . . .''

Connie, who seems to have her husband's number, expresses it simply. "He wanted somebody to play ball with, so he organized a team.''

"Yes,'' Stone continues, "we didn't have anybody to play against, so I took a bus and went around the city of Los Angeles into all the different neighborhoods and organized seven other teams in the city. I was about ten or eleven at that time. The other teams couldn't get balls and bats, so I showed them how to go to the different merchants for sponsorship. Our team's uniform said Black's Butcher Shop. The "uniform'' was a T-shirt and a cap. I used to stand behind the fence at Gilmore Field when the local minor league team worked out. When they hit the ball over the fence, I'd run and get it. Eventually they put a policeman back there and I'd race him for the balls. He'd try and get them away from me but I'd throw them to my brother who was on a bike. He'd ride away and hide them and then come back. We got all the balls that way.''

Stone goes on, obviously delighted with this memory. Like Jim Irwin he has a way of smiling that's disarming. When you least expect it, a small, self-deprecating grin steals quickly across his face. It just as quickly fades, however, and it's back to serious business again. ''Then we'd rummage through their barrels, where they threw away all the broken bats. My father used to nail the bats back together and tape them up. So pretty soon I was collecting enormous numbers of bats and balls. The other teams didn't have enough so I would go around and deliver them.'' He laughs. ''We had eight teams in our league, and I organized all eight so I'd have a place to play. I always was that way even as a kid.'' Tacking on a summarizing thought, he says, ''So I guess the Depression instilled something about the need for financial security but the instincts for organization were always there.''

Connie characterizes her husband in other ways. ''There's just something about your energy level that's different,'' she says. ''Everybody notices it around here that, when you go away for a few days, there's kind of a void, a change in the type of energy. When you get back, BOOM. But it's positive energy. I like it. The days just quicken.''

We have finished our entree and Mary serves us dessert, some kind of a peach concoction. We ask for herb tea and prepare ourselves for further conversation.

I asked if he was still working as hard after he moved to the East, to Boston.

''No,'' Stone answers, and then decides to qualify it. ''For the first two or three years, I was working pretty hard.'' He explains, however, that part of the motive of the move was to slowly alter his pace, not necessarily to move from California. ''My inclination,'' he answers, ''was to slow down, to start doing it gradually.'' Connie remembers that by that time, they had had their first child, and Marty had become ''much more involved in family life.''

As we talk, a whirlwind in sweatshirt, jeans and pigtails blows through the kitchen headed straight for our table and her mother's arms. This is Katie, the Stones' five-year-old daughter. She is experiencing some difficulty in another area of the house that seems to be related to a video cassette player and her older brother. Connie listens to the child's story, offers a few words of advice, strokes her hair and sends her on the way. Katie's father watches the scene, but continues with his dialogue.

"Yes," he says, "I really intended to start slowing down a lot and then finally when we moved up here, I knew I was going to slow down a lot." He suddenly rises from the table and announces, "I'll let you two talk for a second. I've got to go to the john. I'll be back in a flash."

As he gets up to leave, Connie says, "At least he didn't say I'll be back in a flush; he usually does." When I don't see anything particularly significant in that, she adds, "His business at Monogram was toilets." We both laugh.

"How does it work," I asked her. "Does he make the decisions or do you move around him?"

"It's hard to say," she thinks. "Like probably with any couple, you manipulate each other to a certain extent. But I really think we both do make the decisions. Fortunately, we both are generally on the same kind of a wavelength that way. When he wanted to move, my daughter, whom he adopted when we started living together, was nine and I didn't want her being a teenager in Southern California. I think it creates problems that you can't work around. It's too fast. I grew up in the Midwest where you had time to be a child and you had time to be a teenager, had time to sort your life out. So I really felt for that reason I would rather not be in Southern California. It was terrific for me when I was in my twenties. And when I had just a small child, I could take her every weekend and go to the beach. So I was happy about the move. Another reason, which he doesn't say and he didn't even tell me, was he had just gone through a divorce, and my milieu would have been the same friends that he and Elaine had had for twenty-five years. So to equalize it, we moved to Boston." It seems like a logical and yet very caring strategy.

"It was real good thinking," she concludes. "He's incredibly logical always. I mean, really." Connie also admits that one of her husband's essential attributes is his sense of humor. "It's his main saving grace," she says and then she continues with the obvious. "He's real intense, real intense. When we have to make decisions like that, somehow they just evolve. We were going to buy a house and settle down in California and then we went through 'Why California? Why not somewhere else and, if so, where would it be?' And then when we bought the ranch here, it was to be a real estate investment and a second home and we kept coming and we kept realizing that we didn't want to go back there. So we thought, 'If you were going to live where there is cold and winter, you might as well live where you could use the cold and use the winter a lot more.' You can't use it a lot in Boston."

Marty is back, having caught the tail end of our conversation.

"When we lived in Massachusetts it was a lot less frantic. I mean, my office was in the house, not in a building. I spent a lot of time with the kids and a lot of time with the Red Sox.

Connie concedes, "It was an improvement over L.A." Her husband, applying Connie's comparison to standards, says, "I think it was an improvement over ninety percent of the male population, not just L.A." But Connie doesn't agree. "I mean as far as spending time with the kids and the family maybe that's true, but I don't think it is as far as your business days are concerned, because I think your idea of the average . . ." She stops mid-sentence, looks at me and says simply, "For a while it was real hectic. He was at home so it wasn't that kind of running back and forth, but I mean there were seventeen people in the house all the time."

I suggest that the average person with a business on the West Coast doesn't usually pick up and move to the East.

Stone explains, "I was working out of my house mainly so it didn't matter. The ideal place to have operated was New York City. But I didn't want to live in New York City, so we moved to Boston. That's an hour from New York by shuttle and I could still live out in the country and enjoy myself. We were living west of Boston."

Connie amplifies. "Marty lived his whole life in California; he never lived anywhere else. And so he said, 'I want to see what it's like to live in another climate.' " She adds, mockingly. " '. . . before I die.' " We all laugh; I observe that I don't know how she did it.

Connie continues, "I can remember my sister pulling me aside and saying, 'You can't live like this much longer. Every time you come to town, by the time you leave I'm going like this—' " She grimaces and tightens the muscles all over her body.

Stone says he was not aware of this. "No," he says, "as a matter of fact I'm aware of the contrary—the fact that I've slowed up so much."

"But," says Connie, "I think it still exists on a different level."

"You know," her husband responds, "I'm less frenetic than ninety percent of the people I know. When we decided to come here, a lot of our friends thought I was crazy. But you see, I had been changing for eleven years and yet somehow I've continued to work.

"I finally decided," he recalls, "that I was sick and tired of having my office in the corporate office because everybody came in to brownnose or else to build me into their decisions, which I didn't want them to do. I wanted them to make their own decisions. I found I was wasting half of my day by being in a place so obsessive. By officing at home I found I had a huge amount more time for everything—my personal kinds of things, anything I wanted to do. I mean my time just wasn't being wasted in vast amounts. It's true this way I'm on the phone a lot more than I want to be and I have to travel more than I would otherwise have to.''

Although no direct reflection on the Stones, it can become tiring to listen to and read these accounts of feverish activity, of men and women who insist on doing too much in the service of what they characterize as advancement, financial security or in search of a benchmark against which to pace themselves. And to hear spouses complain of tight schedules and lack of awareness. Perhaps the fault lies in the American way of life, at least as interpreted by these individuals. Does one always have to go higher and faster, become richer and richer? Is there satisfaction in that—or only frustration? And what of the people who must gyrate around these spinning tops of activity—the family members? Must success, as defined in the business world, court this kind of self-denial? What can life really be like lived at this pace? Exciting? Fred Rizk came close to saying yes: the goal has become the end in itself. Alan Keiser said work was fun, and when it wasn't, you got out. Can you believe such easily stated opinions? Can this be the same definition of fun as we conventionally know it? Lighthearted, rejuvenating, purposeless.

Applied by the Type A personalities of this book, the definition of fun seems to refer to hard work, endless phone calls, business luncheons and overloaded commitments. As the modern business world seems to interpret it, fun sounds more like days and nights of overwork. Jack Rutta says it requires stubborn intellect. Rizk and Mulhair and Stone speak of control. Seen in this light, you can begin to understand how Martin Stone, an otherwise insightful and intelligent man, could have spent most of his adult life applying the practicalities of business economy to his personal life, convincing himself of the adequacy of statistics, predicting his early death from heart disease and inducing compulsive behavior about diet and exercise that, while reinforcing his concerns, frustrated the happiness of those around him.

Connie says, ''You go in spurts now. I mean the past month you've been real busy and the next month will be busy but then you'll go through a couple of months where you'll calm down for a while.''

I asked if there are any problems adjusting from the peace and quiet of the mountains to the hectic city pace.

''No,'' Stone answers impassively. ''You operate at a much faster pace, and I want it that way because when I go to New York or I go to Los Angeles, I want to get it done with and get back. I'd just as soon get it over with. I schedule everything at once.''

Says Connie, "Oh, when he goes there, it's total reversion."

He agrees with her. "It's just pure chaos." Then he slows down and thinks it out a bit. "Well, it's true. If I go to Los Angeles for five days, the day will be 100 percent booked. I'll have a breakfast meeting, two meetings in the morning, a meeting for lunch, two or three meetings in the afternoon, a dinner meeting and calls all day and driving all over from appointment to appointment. I do that for five days and leave. But I schedule three weeks' worth of meetings and visits in a week because I don't want to be there for three weeks."

"He does that when he goes to New York, too," Connie offers. But Stone quickly changes the subject to get to his point, making use of one of his summarizing statements, which in effect returns us to the beginning of the conversation. "Anyway, I finally went to Pritikin because I was really scared about the continual high cholesterol. And I read Pritikin's first book, which came out probably about '76, '77. And I talked to a lot of my friends from the Beverly Hills Tennis Club who had gone to the Santa Monica center, particularly Max Polansky. I used to play tennis with Max, who had had two bypasses. One day, I played vigorous tennis with him for an hour and a half—singles—and I kept really worrying about him. Finally he said, 'Oh, you don't have to worry at all about me. I went to Pritikin. I feel sensational and this is no problem at all.' "

He pauses and asks Mary for more tea. She delivers it in a steaming mug. "This isn't the stuff I don't like, is it? he asks her. "No," she tells him, "you don't like Red Zinger."

"He doesn't like that," Connie confirms.

"But the more I thought about it," Stone goes on, "I thought about all my friends from the tennis club. And I kept thinking maybe I should go to Pritikin." He pauses to sip his tea, and then he says conclusively, "So I went. When I was admitted to the center, I weighed 196 pounds, which I had always thought was normal for me. I kidded myself about having a massive bone structure. I'm five feet, ten inches, but at 196 nobody said I was fat. I mean I ran thirty miles a week and my exercise level was very heavy. But at Pritikin, my weight went down to about 175. I lost twenty-one pounds in twenty-six days, partly because I misread the exercise prescription and did more than I was supposed to."

Stone says he discovered the food at the center was substantially different than the diet he was used to. "It was a lot different. You see, I didn't understand cholesterol well enough, even with everything I had read. And I still had a lot of fat in my diet, proportionally. I ate a lot of pasta that had oil and garlic on it, although I avoided butter and cream and all that. And I should have known more about the cheeses. I used to have only skim-milk cheeses—which still have a heavy amount of fat. But I thought as long as I had skim-milk cheeses I was fine. So I used a tremendous amount of cheese.

"At the center," he remembers, "I ate everything in sight. I would sit and eat with Nathan once in a while and I ate more than he did. At first it amazed me to look at him eat but then after a while I was eating more than he was. I would go in and have two lunches, two dinners. They'd come around with the two choices of dinners and I'd say I wanted them both. And I'd pick. I'd have a big fresh salad and then a cooked salad of the same size for lunch and then all the bread I could stuff down my throat. I was running seventy-two miles a week, plus doing the aerobics in the middle of the day. But at the end of the twenty-six days," he concludes, "I felt terrific."

Katie runs back into the kitchen again. This time, she heads straight for her father and whispers in his ear. He listens carefully, lowering his voice to her level and offering advice, which she seems to consider valid. After a few minutes, she turns on her heels and heads back to where she came from.

I asked if he enjoyed being at the center.

"Yes," says Marty, "as a matter of fact I liked it."

Connie says, "You thought it would bother you."

He agrees. "It looked kind of dreary and depressing and I thought I'd be around old, sick people, which there were."

Connie adds, "You thought you wouldn't like the confinement."

Her husband doesn't respond to her remark and says, "But I liked the people because all of them had a vigorous interest in life, the kind of people who were unwilling to accept what was happening to them and were going to take responsibility for their own health. Now, I relate very well, especially to people who don't sit back waiting for whatever is going to come along to happen. And most of the people I met were kind of take-charge people. As Connie will tell you, I'm kind of inherently shy, but at the center, I would always go to a different table and sit down with different people and talk to them. It was amazing the stories they all had. There were a lot of very interesting people there who didn't look interesting when you saw their misshapen bodies in their jogging suits and all. And I really had a lot of fun talking to all the people. So the dreariness of the place ceased to bother me."

Connie Stone actively supported her husband's decision to attend the Pritikin Longevity Center in Santa Monica. "I thought it was a really good idea," she says. "I'd lived with him . . ." She stops and starts again, "I mean from the first day we were together, he'd been telling me, 'I'm going to have a heart attack. I probably won't be around long.' So I said, 'Please, go, with my blessing, go.' "

Martin Stone left the Pritikin center, having lost weight and become more informed about the cholesterol that haunted him. The diet served at the center is the primarily vegetarian Regression Diet, and Stone intended to maintain himself on this, rather than the Maintenance Diet, which allows a higher daily ration of animal protein. "I stayed on the Regression Diet for two years," he recalls. "But my cholesterol went right back up to 225, not 275, which it had been, but 225, within a month or two on the Maintenance Diet," he says disgustedly. "Then I called up Pritikin and we had a long talk. He asked me if I was absolutely certain that I was following the Maintenance Diet. I told him, 'Absolutely, I'm following it exactly.' "

Connie interrupts him saying, "He was doing nothing but grazing."

Her husband continues. "Nathan said, 'Well, then, it's conceivable that you need the Regression Diet to hold it down.' And then he said, 'There are people like you. I wouldn't know for sure that's your situation because I don't know for sure what you're eating. But I'd suggest to you that you go back to the Regression Diet.'

"So," Stone says, the tone in his voice suggesting the resignation he must have felt, "I went back to the Regression Diet, as close as I could come to it, bearing in mind that I was eating on airplanes and staying in hotels. But it was somewhere between the Regression Diet and the Maintenance Diet. And my cholesterol for two years stayed between 165 and 190. I was thinking about the fact that Pritikin had said that if you kept it at around 150 for two years, you'd get regression of plaque in the arteries. But what has since happened to me is that I have gradually eroded and gotten worse. I can't stay on the Regression Diet.

"After three years, my cholesterol had gotten back up to around 252. So I went back to Pritikin for two weeks. Then," he says with the satisfaction of having negotiated a lucrative business deal, "I started making an arrangement. Since Monogram's office was only three blocks away from the Santa Monica center, I would call Nathan every time I was going to be in L.A. and I'd say, 'Do you have a closet or some room?' The first time he said, 'Yes, we have this one room that is just so horrible we never rent it out. I hesitate to put anybody in there.' I told him, 'I don't care, as long as I can eat the meals.' So he would let me come and stay there. I used it as a hotel for my trips to Los Angeles. I ate all my meals there. I would even drag my business people there for lunch meetings." He laughs and Connie adds, "Then they'd go and have lunch somewhere else."

"Usually," he explains, "I was in Los Angeles a week at a time, sometimes two weeks. So I just used the center as a hotel, as a place to stay, and all they charged me for was the meals. It also gave me a place to work out. I could go down to the gym and work out or I could use their changing rooms, or use my room as a changing room and run. So I started to stay there, oh, probably four or five times a year for a week at a time, maybe two weeks at a time. This system kept my cholesterol down between 165 and 190. And then time went by and I was staying there less and less and traveling more and more and I couldn't get my cholesterol down; I couldn't keep it down."

"So," says Connie, again directing her comments back to her husband, as if she's thinking it out, "you got so you went back almost once a year and stayed there as a fix." Then she smiles and lets the cat out of the bag. "Because," she says, "you would . . ." She looks at me. "We're talking chocolate chip cookies."

"I would get very discouraged," he admits.

"Sweets?" I asked.

"Yeah," he answers woodenly.

"Always sweets," says Connie. "Because he could care less about anything else."

"Yes," her husband admits, "chocolate chip cookies." Then he adds, to move the conversation along, "But anyway what happened was . . ."

Connie, however, interrupts and offers the information that her husband is a binger when he starts.

"Anyway . . ." Stone begins again.

But Connie still hasn't finished with him. "He doesn't even bother with a cup," she says. "He just takes a spoon into the ice cream."

Her husband doesn't respond, and we are all quiet. Mary comes over with more tea and clears the rest of the dishes off the table.

II

"I didn't believe it at first. It took a couple of months to sink in."

So Martin Stone muddled along, anticipating the fatal heart attack, constantly fighting to keep his cholesterol down and not succeeding as he desired. Life might have continued on that way for the Stones, except for a chance meeting on New Year's Eve in 1981 that opened the door to a small ray of hope. But until that evening, the battle against cholesterol seemed futile.

Stone recalls the dietary changes he made before he entered the Pritikin Center. "I was gradually getting rid of meat altogether," he relates. "I used to think veal had very little fat in it. When I was eating veal I thought I was going just fine. I ate no butter; I peeled the skin off all the chicken. I didn't eat anything fried. I was cutting way down on eggs, but when I did have eggs, I had omelets—cheese omelets. And a cheese omelet is probably the single fattest thing you can eat, of anything that you could pick. So," he summarizes, "I had a smattering of knowledge. My father and I had more knowledge than most people, but not nearly enough. With my constitution, I couldn't keep my cholesterol under 275 even that way. Of course, I didn't realize there was any cholesterol at all in breads or pancakes or any of that stuff.

"That's where I always cheated the most," he says, "ice cream. And I used to assume that if you ate apple pie and cherry pie that that was fine, because they had no fat in them." He laughs at his naivete. "Well," he says in his own defense, "I never understood these other things. I just thought it was fruit, and the crust was like bread, and as long as I didn't eat cream pies or anything like that I was fine." He chuckles and adds, in a manner suggesting the easy sense of humor his wife alludes to, "So I thought . . . so I would eat lemon meringue pies and cherry pies and apple pies."

Stone admits that he was frustrated that his continued efforts to keep his cholesterol down were not yielding the results he desired. "But," he continues, "at The Pointe resort last New Year's Eve, we met this fellow who had been with NIH [National Institutes of Health] and had been involved with the ten-year NIH study on the effects of cholesterol. He had brought in Bob Levy to run that program.

"This man listened to my story and then he said, 'Dr. Levy would see you, I'm sure.' I told him, 'I've really got to find a way to get the cholesterol down.' He said, 'He doesn't take private patients, but I could call him up and arrange for you to see him about this.' So I flew down to New York and I met with Bob and he agreed to accept me as a patient, and I started taking cholestyramine at his suggestion."

A veteran of the NIH study in which drug therapy figured prominently, it was logical that Dr. Levy would have recommended cholestyramine to Martin Stone. It is one of a class of drugs known to be successful in lowering cholesterol. Levy's NIH study, undertaken by the National Institute of Heart, Blood and Lung, conclusively linked the lowering of serum cholesterol to reduction in the incidence of heart disease. Although patients were told to watch their diets, the primary treatment utilized in the study was drug therapy. The study is generally considered of particular significance, however, because it was the first to document conclusively the direct correlation between high cholesterol and heart disease, an issue that has been debated in the medical establishment for years.

"Now Levy told me," says Stone, " 'You've got to remember that it gives a lot of people gas and constipation, although we don't know of any dangerous side effects.' Nathan said later this was nonsense, that it can cause liver disease."

Because drug side effects can vary from patient to patient, drug therapy for high cholesterol is usually prescribed only after other methods have not proved effective, as appears to be the case with Martin Stone.

"I solved the problem of constipation," Stone recalls, "by taking bran. I'd been taking bran regularly anyhow and I doubled the dose. Levy was fascinated with that and I started to give him regular statements of what I was eating and how much bran I was taking. Soon I was using three packets of the stuff instead of the six they recommend, and it got my cholesterol down very quickly from about 225 or 235 to about 190.

"And I was not having constipation or anything," he continues. "When I told Nathan about it, he was furious. I had confided to Levy that I regarded Nathan as the most important pioneer in this whole field of cholesterol in American history. Levy was always very diplomatic, but you could tell he was very upset at me for saying that. But I went further. I said, 'You know what your study does is confirm Nathan Pritikin's work, only you're afraid to confine it to diet.' In answer, Levy gave me a whole series of reasons why they couldn't do it with diet."

I asked Stone whether he had been under the care of another doctor at the time.

"Yes," he answers. "Jerry Port in Beverly Hills. Jerry didn't think I should really be that worried about my condition." (Dr. Port's records indicate that during the period running from 1970 to 1974, Martin Stone's cholesterol hovered around 250.)

"Then," says Connie, moving the story along and directing her remarks to her husband, "the only problem we had after that was that you realized you were starting to use the cholestyramine as a crutch." He nods in agreement.

"So he could cheat more," she explains. "That worried him." Then switching gears, she says, "You know, you would eat a bag of

chocolate chip cookies and then have six packets of cholestyramine.''
She turns back to me, "So he asked to quit the cholestyramine.''

Stone takes up the story. "Finally,'' he says with a sigh, like a
climber who has passed all the obstacles but has not yet reached the top
of the mountain, "one of my hiking buddies, Dick Handler, suggested
that I take a heart catheterization—an angiogram. He said to me, 'You
can't go on living such a stressed life over this issue.' His remarks got
me to thinking about it. Jim Fixx had just died, and that bothered me.
I'd called Nathan about that. Nathan's opinion was that it was crazy for
anybody to do the kind of stressful exercise Jim Fixx did while still on
the typical American diet and without a stress test.''

He pauses for a minute, the room is silent, except for the pasta-
maker Mary has plugged in and is feeding dough through. The next
sentence comes easily and in that curious summarizing manner Stone
has when speaking, especially about weighty topics. "So it was then I
decided to have a heart catheterization.''

Sitting up in her seat, Connie continues the saga, remembering
details. "After he made that decision, I asked Marty, 'What kind of
blockage do you think you'll get?' '' She pauses and looks me straight
in the eye, as if to emphasize what she's going to say. "You know what
he said? He said, 'Eighty to eighty-five percent.' ''

"I thought in at least one vessel,'' her husband says and then adds,
almost to himself, "that's what I thought I would have. I thought that,
because my cholesterol continued to be high, except for that one
two-year period when it was very low, I would have at least eighty
percent blockage in that one artery.''

Connie interjects, "And maybe more you said.''

"And maybe more,'' he agrees.

"You said,'' she reminds him, "you were sure.''

But the story has further to go. Stone decides to describe the
details. "Anyway, I was on one of our hikes up here with a doctor who
used to be an intern with a fellow named Sosa at Albany Medical Center.
Sosa had worked at the Cleveland Clinic when they developed the heart
catheter. This fellow—my hiking friend—said to me that Sosa was the
best on the East Coast. He told me, 'If I were going to have it done
here, that's where I would have it.' I thought about that and then I
called Ted Diethrich at the Arizona Heart Institute [Dr. Edward B.
Diethrich] and I said, 'Ted, I was going to come out and have you do it,
but I think I'm going to do it close to home. And it's been recommended that I go to a guy named Sosa.' Diethrich said he understood
that he was very good. So I said, 'I'm going to have it done that
way.' '' Concluding this aspect of the story, Martin Stone says impas-

sively, "And I went last October to the Albany Medical Center and had the thing done."

I asked Connie if she supported that. "Oh yes," she beams, "you bet."

Before she can say anymore, her husband says, "Well, I examined all the risks and I talked to people about the percentage of danger . . ."

She doesn't let him finish, however. "And I figured with that risk, the knowledge, one way or another . . . it would not be just an unknown. I thought a known quantity in anything was better than the other."

"I was so certain that I would have blockage," says Stone, "that I couldn't believe the test. The doctor said, 'I really would prefer to study it all over and take films of it.' But I could see while he was doing it, so I asked him, 'Why, what do you see?' He said to me, 'Well, I see one narrowing at one point and nothing else.' " Stone pauses, the room is still again, the heavy Adirondack air seems to fill the house and deafen our senses. Connie doesn't say anything and her husband continues. "He went back and he found the narrowing was a kink in the artery where it comes down like that." He loops his fingers around to explain what he's talking about.

"Then he called Dick—the guy who had recommended him in the first place—and he said to him, 'Richard, I don't understand this. I've showed it to all the people around here, too. They don't understand it.' " He pauses for effect. " 'That man has nothing in his arteries. He has totally clear arteries. There's this kink in there at the point where the right descending artery goes at the right angle, which is not likely to cause any problem, although that's the place where stuff will build up. But,' he said, 'at this point he has no congestion in his arteries at all. I've never seen an adult male with a history of high cholesterol, ever, with totally clean arteries.' " Stone concludes with a flourish, still proud of the news.

"Then Sosa called me up and asked me what I had been doing. 'Describe your diet to me,' he said. And I started to tell him about Pritikin. He asked about it and I told him the whole story."

Connie has been listening to all of this, watching her husband, her elbow on the table and her arm bent so that she holds her chin in her hand. There is relief in her eyes. "He said you had the cleanest arteries he had ever seen of any adult . . ." she reminds him.

"Of any man my age," her husband corrects her. He said, " 'I've never seen a fifty-six-year-old man with totally clean arteries.' "

There is a significant lapse in the conversation. Neither seems inclined to offer further editorializing on the effects of the angiogram, each, perhaps, for different reasons. To Connie Stone, the news must have had a great liberating effect. Despite listening closely to her, it's difficult to detect the emotion under her well-chosen words, and because of this, it's more difficult to empathize with the burden she must have carried. To her husband, the news seems to have been ambivalent. For a man as goal-directed as he, the results of the angiogram must have confirmed the wisdom of his conscientious strategies. On the other hand, you wonder if the results offered any insight about his former behavior.

Connie is the first to speak. "I didn't know," she says, "whether to be . . ." But although she is ready to explore this thought further, her husband is thinking along an entirely different track. "So Richard Handler went on the diet—the guy who had recommended Albany Medical Center and recommended the angiogram and who had pooh-poohed Pritikin all the time." He laughs in triumph.

Connie falls in line with what he's saying. "For two years they had this controversy going. Ever time they hiked, they'd argue over it."

"He'd say, 'Pritikin is nothing but a shyster; that's a bunch of bunk to tell people that they can regress plaque in their arteries.' Now," Stone chuckles, "he's on the diet. He bought the Pritikin books and read them all. He's got his wife cooking that way. And that's after telling me that Pritikin was a shyster."

Her husband's points made, Connie continues to evaluate her own response to the news. She says, "And I didn't know whether to be just totally, thoroughly relieved like I'd never been in my life. Or," she pauses and her voice takes on a sharpness, "to be furious when I thought of all those years."

I ask Stone what he thought.

Connie answers for him, "He didn't believe it for a while; it didn't sink in."

He agrees. "It took a long while," he says with classic understatement.

"It was hard to admit," Connie concedes. "His oldest son called me and told me about it, and I said, 'Isn't it great?' I was just on this huge high and he said, 'I think he's slightly disappointed.'"

But her husband isn't having any of this. He backs into one of his concluding statements: "Anyway, I then called Nathan and I asked him how this could be. And Nathan said, 'Well, you did regress with the diet and maybe your tissues have so much cholesterol in them that even though you eat very modest amounts of additional cholesterol, you're still pouring cholesterol from your tissues into your blood stream, which makes your blood levels high.''

"But how did all of this affect you?'' I pushed.

He moves in his chair to get comfortable again, his elbow leaning on the chair's arm, his hands folded. The light outside grows dimmer, seeming to mesh with our mood. He says, "Gradually now I've noticed that I do things without worrying about them or thinking about them. Like I almost never went on one of our long hikes without expecting that one of these days they were going to leave me at the top of the mountain.'' Again the room becomes quiet, even Mary's pasta-maker has quit. "And now,'' he completes the sentence, "I don't think about that.''

"Even after Pritikin,'' says Connie, "up until last October, when he had . . .''

"Because I never felt like I kept it down low enough,'' her husband interrupts. "I fought and fought and fought but I couldn't ever keep it down enough.''

Connie, tightening again, relives a memory. She puts her hands on the table and leans forward, pressing on her elbows. She says, "He used to tell me that might happen to him—that they might have to leave him at the top of the mountain. But then he'd say, 'I suppose that's the way I'd really like to go, you know.' '' She slams the table with her fist, in mock desperation.

But Stone continues to expound on his point. "So anyway,'' he continues, "now I don't think about that as much anymore and I haven't had a blood test since.'' The room breathes again, but he's not ready to let that thought go. "I probably should,'' he muses, "because probably I should continue the same habits. I'm eating in a relatively careful fashion. Except when I travel, I'm not as careful as I used to be.''

The Annenberg School of Communication at the University of Southern Calfornia has recently completed a study of adherence to the Pritikin Program. The research concluded that the difference between strict adherents to this change in life-style and the backsliders who are unable to maintain it lies in the essential strong support of family members, friends and workmates. Without this supportive network, backsliding is predictable. The report concludes with the recommendation that Pritikin Program training should include education of the spouse or loved one, and where that is impossible, people about to embark on this type of dietary and exercise change should be taught strategies for involving significant other members of their immediate environment with their plan.

Gradually, this is becoming Connie Stone's story. From a relatively quiet anecdotal role at the beginning of our conversation, she now emerges as a central character. In this case, however, it is not simply a matter of the level of her support. The emotion that both have avoided thus far in telling their story is beginning to surface.

I wondered how her husband now handles the Pritikin Program on a daily basis.

"I've already crossed that bridge a long time ago," he says. "I don't look upon it as one more day or anything like that. It's a whole lifetime. I'm committed to eating that way and to that level of exercise and trying to manage the stressfulness of my life. I'm committed to that as a way of life and so I don't think about it. That's just the way I assume I eat." He slaps the table lightly. "So," he continues, "this isn't a diet to me; it's nothing that's a temporary thing. I don't really have that much deviation. It's just that I'm aware of any single instance of deviation so I'm bothered by it. I feel much better on those occasions when I'll go four-five days where I'll eat perfectly, when I just won't eat a single thing that's not on the Regression Diet."

He admits that he becomes anxious when he falls off the diet. "When I get off the diet, it does bother me a little bit. I feel guilty for having gotten off the wagon, but I don't really have any doubt that I'll get back on again. I could never go back to eating the diet I used to eat."

"I couldn't either," claims Connie. Her remark is surprising because I remember Marty telling me a few years ago how difficult it was to be on the diet when the rest of the family wasn't having any of it. He had sounded very discouraged.

"I can't envision eating eggs," he says. And then adds, in a voice that tries to be light but nonetheless winces with frustration, "The problem is chocolate chip cookies. I still have a serious weakness and I give in periodically, not nearly as much, however, as I kick myself for. And in terms of stress management, my main thing is giving myself more time between appointments. If I have to be somewhere in a half-hour and I know it takes twenty-five minutes to drive there, instead of leaving twenty minutes ahead of time with twenty-five minutes to go, I'll leave thirty-five minutes ahead so I have ten minutes extra. That's where I get the most stressed—time . . ."

"Or," says Connie, "inconvenience, like having to wait, having to stand in line, having our plane reservations screwed up. But you do it much less than you used to."

From her previous comment, I detected that the Pritikin Program is new to Connie Stone. I asked her if she's been on the diet all along.

"No," she answers, simply, an answer that suggests further implications.

"How did you find it without Connie?" I pressed her husband.

"It was very hard," he answers. "It's easier now. Mostly it's easier for the cook than it is for me. I mean, if Mary had to cook the standard American diet for Connie and then the Pritikin diet for me . . . it was twice as hard."

"But," Connie says, "that's what we did up until last October. We cooked the same things, at some point stopping the process, taking his out and then adding some cheese."

I asked Connie why she had decided to change her eating habits.

"Because from last February until October, even though I hadn't really changed my eating habits, which weren't good . . ." She stops and adds the comfortable yardstick, "but they weren't terrible by most American standards either. They were probably average. And swimming a mile a day, five or six days a week, I gained some weight. And I could feel it. I could feel the difference. There were some extraordinary physiological changes that were going on in my body."

When I wondered that she didn't go on the Pritikin diet to begin with, she makes a dim sound with her breath and admits, "When I look back on it now—and we haven't even talked about it—because it's only occurred to me in the last month or two . . ." She pauses, moves around in her chair and finally comes out with it. "Probably it was anger and resentment. It was almost a weapon to say . . . to deny the whole thing. Like saying, 'Well, I'm not going to do it. Look what I'm eating.' "

Stone breaks in, "I'm going to eat all this shit and I'm going to be alive long after . . ."

Connie acknowledges, "It was maybe cutting off my nose, but on the other hand it . . ."

"It made it much harder for me," he says.

"It was a process I had to go through," Connie makes an attempt to explain. "Then I came to the conclusion that I should do it for my own good. Not just because of the weight but because . . ."

She stops and pokes at a bagel thin her husband has put in front of her. As we have talked, Mary has been slicing and cooking bagels in the oven. Thin like this and crisp from a quick toasting, they taste like cookies. Stone has jumped up, grabbed a handful and brought them back to the table for us. He munches away on his peacefully and listens to his wife. "The scare for me is not like his," she says. "People in my family have had cancer, and I truly believe it helps prevent cancer of the colon and things like that, in addition to the weight and the conditioning. And the truth of the matter is, after I was on it, I felt much better, immeasurably better. I would never go back.''

Understanding her remark, I asked her husband how he coped with being the odd man out at his own table. "Well, it was hard," he answers. "That was not easy."

"We made it always accessible to him and he always had a Pritikin meal," says Connie, sensing what's to come.

I ventured that it is generally important to have the support of the people around you to help with staying on the diet. "You almost were not supportive," I suggested to Connie. This hits a chord. "That's not true," she says testily. But it has also struck something in her husband; he challenges her immediately. "Oh, it is true, Connie. Oh, no, it was totally true."

"I thought that you should . . ."

But he doesn't let her finish: "You thought I should, but you made it murder for me to stay on it."

"Just because I wasn't on it?" she asks him.

"You filled the house with all kinds of things . . ." he accuses.

"That's not true," she repeats.

"Oh, Connie," he drawls at her, grabbing another bagel thin.

"Compared to the average family . . ."

"Your diet compared to the average diet was horrible . . ."

"No, it wasn't."

"And that's why you gained twenty pounds. One time," he confides, "with the cook, I just took a week's worth of her eating and it was disastrous. She put Bailey's Irish Cream in her coffee. She had the worst shit imaginable that she ate and she filled the house . . ."

"That's not true, my computer . . ."

"With cakes, candies, ice cream, cookies. And she said, 'I can't deprive everybody in this household just because of you.' ''

"I was angry," Connie admits, turning to me, "but he's exaggerating."

"I'm not exaggerating," Stone insists.

Connie retreats to her standards, "But it wasn't filled like the average American home."

Her husband laughs thinly but refuses to let up. "We are in total disagreement on that recollection."

Connie, however, wants to pursue it. "There was plenty that was not on his diet," she explains tersely. "On the other hand, there's still stuff in the house for the kids. It's not junk, however, and we go to great lengths to try and improve their diet. But I still feel that, should I decide that I wanted to eat that [conventional American] diet for my own personal something, I should have the right to do that. And I do have the right to do that, and I would do it again.''

He says, ''I didn't stop you from eating it.''

''You didn't,'' she agrees. ''No, and I didn't stop you. And we had a cook that did the Pritikin thing.'' The residue of years of frustration seems to be slowly emerging. ''I mean,'' she says, ''I was angry but I still feel that if he felt that strongly that heart disease was going to kill him, if he really believed that, it was up to his own discipline not to eat it.'' And then deftly and unexpectedly, she brings up the heavy ammunition. ''Because when I wouldn't have it in the house, he would go out and get it. He'd go to the lawyer's office—who had cookie stashes and he would get them. And I thought, 'Well, it's a personal decision.' And I still feel that way.''

In response to Connie's revelation, Stone closes the subject, ''I will not comment further on that issue.''

Before she gives in, however, Connie consolidates her position. ''But if he had had a heart attack,'' she explains, ''I might not have responded that way. If he had had a heart attack—I've thought about that often—I would have been so fanatical that I would probably have hired some little person to follow him around and grab fat out of his mouth if he tried to eat any. But having not had one, it was different.''

After he completed the angiogram and accepted its results, Martin Stone says that the agony of living with the certainty of a heart attack has left him. ''On the other hand,'' he says, qualifying his words, ''I still am concerned about my cholesterol and want to keep it down. The idea of the immediacy of a heart attack has left me. It took a long while to wear off but it wore off. So I don't really think about that. I haven't even taken a blood test since then and I used to take them once a month or once every two months for the cholesterol.''

Connie remembers, ''He got so good at it that he could always tell, give or take five, where his cholesterol was. Because he feels it.''

''I can normally tell you what my pulse and blood pressure are too,'' Stone contends. ''I can sense it.''

I wanted to know if he had thought about whether it might be worse to have the experience of a heart attack and know that you're a heart patient or to live the way he's lived for so long. ''I don't know,'' he answers, ''but, you know, it did something else that's probably pretty good.''

Connie laughs. She's heard it before. ''He's an optimist,'' she says, "absolutely. 'It's raining on our picnic? Well, at least there won't be any ants.' "

"No," he says seriously, disliking our frivolity and expanding a thought previously expressed, "I think when you expect that you're not going to live a long life or very much longer, then you really demand better quality for your life. You tend to push out of it the annoyances you would normally just put up with because you don't value time that much. But I got to the point where I valued time immensely. So I would not waste a lot of time going to meetings that I didn't want to go to, or gatherings or just simply spending social time with people I didn't want to."

Connie offers a thought of her own. "I think with the kids was the only time I saw it being fearful for you. He'd look at them sometimes," she explains reflectively, "and say things like, 'Oh, I wonder what Sam will be like when he's twelve. I probably won't be around when he . . .' "

Stone contends that he has no emotional awareness of such thoughts. "Well, I don't know," he says dryly. "I had accepted it for so long I just assumed that this was the way it was going to be." Then he adds, a little irritated by my suggestion, "No, I am not detached from my feelings." But Connie is prepared to take slight issue with this. "You have the ability, though," she says tentatively, avoiding running against the issue head-on, "to look at things very logically that I can't, that I don't think other people can."

"But if it's something you've lived with for a long time . . ." he begins.

However, a thread seems to have snapped inside Connie. "On that subject," she maintains haltingly, "I think you were more detached than I believe anybody could be. I mean I wouldn't be able to sit and look at our kids and say, 'Gee, it's too bad I'm not going to see them grow up.' "

"I didn't say that," her husband answers.

"Yes, you did."

"No," he insists, "I didn't really say that. I never accepted it as certainty. I just thought there was a high probability, a pretty high percentage chance." He repeats himself, "But not a certainty by any means. I never assumed that it was certain." Connie is silent, her breath making a sort of restless, scurrying sound. Unchallenged, Marty continues. "And I think it's since I've accepted the fact that a heart attack isn't imminent I've relaxed a lot about that sort of stuff, a tremendous amount. At first I didn't because people kept asking, 'Why aren't you jubilant?' Well, I knew I should be but I couldn't really feel it yet. I couldn't really believe it. You know, I had called Pritikin and I talked to other people. It just didn't seem logical." Reflectively he adds the ultimate crescendo: "It flew in the face of all that was logical."

Connie adds with a sigh, "After all those years of convincing all of us."

Stone repeats his thought, "I couldn't accept the fact that it was valid. But then gradually I did." Having established that fact, however, he acknowledges he will probably have another angiogram sometime in the future. " 'Cause I would still worry," he explains, "that with a relatively high cholesterol for ten or more years, it could build back, it could build up. I don't know, but at least I'm out from under that cloud."

Connie says, "We look at other people—who was it we were talking about not long ago? His blood pressure is high, his cholesterol was such and such and he has a family history of heart disease. People looking at that kind of thing are more accepting of the fact that something's probably going to happen. But most people—unlike Marty—especially at a young age, don't start doing something about it, start taking control of their lives. They do it after the fact."

"But everything about my life I anticipate," her husband reminds her.

Connie picks up on his idea, and her words have the hollow ring of familiarity. "Control," she says to him, "having things under control and being able to do things that you are able to control."

"Well, I always have looked ahead and anticipated," he muses. "I think that's one of my greatest strengths in business. I've looked beyond the next move—three, four, five, six moves forward—and tried to control each of the subsequent moves so that the ultimate objective could be obtained or avoided. As regards my health, the ultimate objective was to live a long, healthy life. And not to have it end in a quick heart attack at some early point. And all my life, in everything I did, I tried to control my own destiny, so I wasn't willing to just sit back and let these things happen to me."

Listening to Stone's conversation, I'm reminded of Alan Keiser's image of sitting in the chair waiting to die and how that remembrance remains a continued source of motivation for him.

"Marty sees those images ahead of time," confides Connie.

"Well," he responds, "it's not images. I just see results that I want to avoid." He pauses, thinks a moment. "I want to avoid that. I really want to avoid incapacity at all costs. But that in and of itself taught me a lot about how you feel about life when it's about to be taken away. And it's something of the same thing, only different degrees in terms of how I looked ahead at life with the idea of a heart attack hanging over me.'' Although Stone concedes that he was concerned about both an early and unheralded death and incapacity, he says, ''I dread the idea of incapacity, particularly now with a five-year-old and nine-year-old. I think it's very important that I live at least till they're fifteen or sixteen.''

I asked why those particular ages.

''With a boy,'' he replies forcefully, ''I don't think he really needs his father after about fourteen. I think the father has to get out of the boy's way when the boy gets into his mid-teenage years and let him develop.''

''Well,'' laughs Connie, ''maybe a few years before that you could start eating cookies.''

He ignores her comment. ''But Kate's five; she's the younger one.''

''What's left before Martin Stone decides to eat his cookies?'' I asked.

''Well, you know, I really want to spend a lot of time with my kids,'' he begins. ''I want to see them grow up and . . . I just don't know right now. I enjoy doing a lot of things and I enjoy starting up new ventures, and I don't know in advance what ventures they'll be. I do have a feeling—my father was a lot like this. He felt the greatest experiences he could have were learning experiences, and he was just a nut for learning new things. I think I'm somewhat that way. For instance I really want to learn now about different places in the world, not as a tourist, but as a participant. That's what World Paper means to me. I can go to those places and at least to some extent participate in the things that are going on there. So I can get a little deeper into it. So for me World Paper is a learning experience. That's its main function.'' (World Paper is a supplement to regular newspapers now available only in Europe. It's focus is sociopolitical reporting on major issues facing various countries of the world.)

''The thing,'' he continues, ''that has always made me able to walk away from a loss has been the fact that I've regarded it as a learning experience. Whether you make or lose money, you've learned something. You've involved yourself in something exciting. You've done something exciting and interesting even though it may not have turned out well or you may have lost money.''

Connie breaks in. She says to him, ''And the actual money isn't that important to you. It's a way of counting. When the economy was pretty bad a few years ago, '72, I can remember you saying, 'If it goes down because of such and such and such and such, I might lose everything, but I can do it over again. I just don't particularly want to do it now that I'm over fifty.' "

Martin Stone freely admits that he enjoys having money. "It makes it possible to live where I want to live in the style that I want to live. I mean I couldn't live up here if I didn't have access to an airplane."

"And," says Connie, "we vitally love this place."

"Yes," he counters. "This place takes a fortune to maintain."

Connie adds her opinion about the value of money. "Money makes it easy to stay on the diet. It makes life easy. The practical things—you don't want to have to spend time cleaning your house? Why should you have to spend time cleaning your house if you don't have to."

Stone continues, "It enables me to get into something like World Paper. I'd never have been able to do anything like that."

"There are a lot of people who have money," says Connie, "who are so busy just making the money that they really don't enjoy it."

Considering his various experiences both with conventional medicine and its alternatives, I asked Martin Stone if he had any opinions about the state of the medical profession.

"Well, I think it's much too dogmatic," he answers. "I think all professions are much too dogmatic. They breed that, because there's a fixed body of learning. Oh, it changes a little here and there at the periphery, but you get through law school and the bar exam by memorizing or learning this fixed body of knowledge and your mind gets surrounded. I often said the more college a person has the less creativity is left in him. Now, I think you can depart your own field and go to another field and become very creative, but it's harder. The more training you have in your own field the harder it is to be creative in it. Then we all tend to get so caught up in degrees and certificates. That's why Pritikin wasn't accepted by the medical profession. He wasn't a doctor. And if he'd done the same things he did and had only been an MD . . ."

We've finished our stash of bagels, so he gets up for more. The rest of his sentence is lost as he moves to the other part of the kitchen. This newest batch of bagel thins is different from the first. I suggest that with these around he doesn't need chocolate chip cookies. Immediately he picks up on my thought. "You know," he shouts to Mary, crunching away, "if you put some chocolate chips in these things . . ." We all laugh, even Mary.

"I'd like to see the medical profession expanded through interaction with chemists, physicists, with people who are in research disciplines,'' he says as he distributes the new bagels. ''We tend to be captive to our own training.''

Based on his experiences in the contemporary American business world, I wondered if he had an opinion about whether it fosters inevitably adverse effects on a person's health. Martin Stone takes immediate issue with the idea. ''I don't think it has anything to do with health,'' he says. ''I would bet you that on the whole businessmen are in as good health as any other profession or group of people.'' I look at him skeptically and he continues, trying to convince me. ''I think it's just the American way of life,'' he says. ''I think that our problem is that we overbook our time, therefore we have to do things like grab fast foods. We don't have time to prepare foods, and you can't be on a good diet if you don't prepare the food. I mean, what are you going to do? Order something delivered, like a pizza or fried chicken or stop at McDonald's?''

The idea builds. ''I don't think it's the business way of life. I don't think it's extra pressure in that way of life versus anything else. We book our time 108 percent, and that makes it impossible to live without unnecessary stress. It makes it impossible to do a lot of things—take the time to spend with the kids, take the time to prepare food, take the time to do a lot of things that are important in life. I think it's what happens to all of us in any way of life. I would guess business people are in as good condition and live as long as, say, teachers.''

''You think their stress levels are the same?'' asks Connie.

''I think their stress levels are the same.''

''Do you think the blue-collar worker . . .'' she starts to ask, but he cuts her off.

''I think there are lots of different kinds of stress. There are certain kinds of stress that I think are harmful. There is another type of stress that not only do I not think is harmful, but I think the overall impact on you is probably beneficial.''

I asked him if he considered himself a Type A personality. ''I believe,'' he says tentatively, ''in that to a certain extent.'' But Connie says, ''I see you as kind of a reformed A—that you go off the wagon once in a while but then you recognize it when you do and you get into a kind of negative stress.''

He doesn't respond to her viewpoint, but continues to enlighten his own proposition. ''I think,'' he says, ''there's a certain amount of stressful life involvement that when you lose that, you shorten your life. It's what happens to people when they retire. There's a certain amount of stress that goes with multiple human relationships and contacts and the tensions of business situations. When you lose those, you lose that edge and excitement. And I think people tend to atrophy. Their soul atrophies like a muscle, and they die.'' It's an interesting image. ''They die much earlier than they would otherwise die. So I think a certain amount of stress and tension and hubbub is necessary to life and to long life. I think longevity is actually aided and added to by certain types of stress.

''Well, all types of human relationships involve stress. All types of business relationships involve stress. It's what you've learned to deal with and are comfortable with, but it's still stressful. And I think if it stresses you in a comfortable way, it's beneficial—the same way as you stress your heart muscle when you exercise. But if you stress the heart more than you ought to or in quick sudden bursts, it's harmful.

''Now,'' he continues, ''while it's beneficial to stress yourself, you can overdo it. And when you overstress yourself, it's the same thing as overstressing your heart physically. So you have to determine what kind of stress is comfortable to you in terms of your being able to deal with it, both heart-wise and otherwise. I think the same thing is true of your mind and your whole psyche—that you should stress yourself mentally for maximum benefit to yourself. Just as you should stress your heart regularly for maximum benefit to your heart. It's true of all the muscles, it's true of the leg muscles, the arm muscles, the heart muscle, and I think it's actually true of your mind. And I think it's true of your heart, your soul.''

It's a poetic thought, well constructed. It lingers in the air like a sweet scent. As the three of us sit and savor it, young Katie bursts into the kitchen again to where we are sitting. This time there are tears in her eyes. She melts into her father's arms and he asks her to explain what's bothering her. The problem comes out in bursts of incomplete sentences. ''It can't be that bad,'' he says. But, for Katie, it is. He asks his wife, ''What's going on here?''

''Well,'' Connie answers sagely, ''it's been rainy and they've been inside all day.''

''All right,'' he says, ''let's go see what's going on.'' Martin Stone gets up from the table, a couple of bagel thins in one hand, his child's small wrist in the other. He heads out to search out the culprit to put things to rights. A household scene just like that of any other, enacted in thousands of homes across the country every day. But here, after everything that's been said, after everything that's been experienced, there's a certain poignancy to it. And you think to yourself—as you watch Katie and her father stroll out of the kitchen together—you're glad Martin and Connie Stone are finally able to enjoy it.

Epilogue

"By 1985, half the people in this country will be on my diet."

I first met Nathan Pritikin in 1980, when a friend called and asked if I would accept an assignment to interview Pritikin for a local Southern California magazine. I'd been following Nathan, intrigued by both his dietary recommendations and the explicit implication of his program—that people should take responsibility for their health. I won't say that I jumped at the assignment; I had heard some pervasive rumors about how difficult and unpredictable Pritikin could be. Eventually, however, I decided to give it a try.

The first roadblock was establishing a date and time for the interview. Mr. Pritikin, I was told, "was just too busy."

"How busy can he be?" I asked. "Well," began the well-meaning PR person, "he gets up at six o'clock and by six-thirty he's on the treadmill and then he goes for his morning run, and then there's breakfast and then he speaks to his groups."

"Fine," I said, "plug me in."

"What?" came the sounds of questioned disbelief from the other end of the line.

"Plug me in to whatever he's doing," I repeated. "I'll just go along with him."

My less-than-eager contact stuttered and stammered her way through a few additional sentences but finally agreed to my suggestion for an interview-on-the-fly. I guess I should have sensed on the day of our interview a few weeks later—as I walked with Nathan on the treadmill and ran with him down the same route thousands of center participants have also traveled—that working with Nathan Pritikin would be an unpredictable adventure.

But I didn't. I was, nonetheless, suitably enough impressed with the content of our conversation that day that I later accepted an offer to work in the Pritikin organization. What Pritikin said made sense to me, although in many aspects I took issue with how he said it. My hunch was that if Nathan's message could be suitably refined so that it had value not only for heart patients but for the great majority of people interested in preventive medicine, we might really be on to something. The inside gossip implied that a small shove in the right direction was all that was needed, that Nathan wanted to do things correctly, but just didn't have the time to figure out what that meant.

The gossip was wrong, and so was I. Nathan Pritikin was a man with a vision he had no desire to compromise. He believed in his program and had no inclination to refine it. This, in and of itself, was an essential element of Nathan's differences with the medical establishment. Nathan's methods were directly antithetical to those of scientists and medical researchers working in the area of nutrition and degenerative disease. These individuals had been trained, as I was, in the scientific method. Summarized briefly, the methodology proceeds as follows. One starts with a premise he would like to investigate. First a literature search is undertaken, to see what others have done in this area and to offer insight into the precise nature of the research possibilities that present themselves. This accomplished, hypotheses are formulated, questions that might be tested. These are narrowed down to only one. (There may be additional sub-hypotheses, but the search always begins with one. If you can't define your interests or problems in terms of one major hypothesis, you are advised to go back and rethink your problem.) This established, you proceed to design your study in order to prove or disprove your hypothesis, defining your sample type and size, data collection, as well as the methods by which to compute the statistical significance of what you collect. Next you proceed to conduct your study and evaluate your results and their implications. Depending on what you find, you may call it a day, or as is more usually the case, proceed back to from whence you began, formulating more hypotheses, completing further testing and so on.

Nathan Pritikin remained satisfied with having implemented the first two steps of the scientific method. He reviewed the literature and developed one fundamental hypothesis: That a high complex–carbohydrate, lowfat, low-cholesterol diet would help in controlling heart disease. He proceeded to utilize his hypothesis, unshackled by the burden to prove it scientifically. The proof, he always felt, was evident in his improved health and that of the thousands of people who had elected to follow his example. What research he did publish was primarily descriptive, following selected patients for limited periods of time. Scientific research, however, deals in what is verifiable, over long periods of time and in representative populations. To Nathan, this was all too much folderol. He wanted to get things done.

Nathan. Everyone called him that. His secretary answered the phone with a more formal, "Mr. Pritikin's office," but as soon as he picked up the receiver, it was Nathan. Nathan, a small man physically, but with a big idea that became a national awareness.

Months after my magazine interview, when I had bitten the bullet and gone to work for Nathan Pritikin, I put myself on an airplane, the object of which was to visit the known authorities in the area of degenerative disease and nutrition. I wanted to know what they thought and where Nathan stood with them. That way I would have a better idea of what my challenges would be. I went to Dallas to visit Dr. Scott Grundy, director of the Center for Human Nutrition at the University of Texas Health Science Center; to Framingham to visit Dr. William Castelli; to Stanford, to speak with Dr. John Farquhar, director of the Stanford Heart Disease Prevention Program, and his committed staff; to heart disease researcher Dr. William Haskill, also at Stanford; to the Harvard University School of Public Health; even to visit Kenneth Cooper—the exercise guru—in Dallas.

The Program received, as they say in show business, mixed reviews. Generally favorable opinions about the validity of his theory were often somewhat mitigated by the persona of Nathan Pritikin himself—a nonmedical man, interfering in the well-ordered business of medicine. And there was also the issue of commerciality.

Nathan seemed to be playing an extremely precarious game— endangering the potential positive reception of his program by setting himself up as a business enterprise. Depending on whom you talked to, this was more or less of a problem. The academicians, whose environment was the predictable world of intellectual thought, tended to be more concerned about this issue than independent researchers whose intuition and research had led them to conclusions not dissimilar from Nathan's. All, however, agreed with the need for verifiable research results and some felt that the captive audience of the Pritikin centers was a ready-made population for long-term research projects that would investigate, and hopefully substantiate once and for all, Nathan's claims.

One additional aspect of Pritikin's public profile often confounded people: his tendency to unilaterally apply his theory to the major health problems confronting modern society, from heart disease to cancer. The issue was not necessarily that he was wrong, but that he should not speak until he had "proof."

I came back from my brief tour with three conclusions. First, that Nathan was definitely on to something in his opinions about the relationship between diet and life-style and heart disease, and that the "major figures" supported his approach, although publicly they weren't necessarily ringing any bells about it. Second, that the challenges of preventive medicine are infinitely more complicated than I had previously understood and Nathan was prepared to acknowledge. Third and finally, that Nathan's message—the way he insisted on communicating it—was a publicist's nightmare.

Nathan Pritikin was a maverick—a zealot, as Martin Stone once characterized him—even a fanatic. But that suited Nathan just fine. I always sensed he liked being on the outside looking in; it gave him more power, power he wouldn't have had if he had been an insulated member of the establishment. He had work to do and he wanted to get it done. "People are dying," he used to tell me when I'd sit with him, attempting to interest him in schedules and plans. "We can't wait." Plans held no truck with Nathan. He may not have known his audience as well as he hoped, but he was buoyed by the impact of his program for people who had experienced it firsthand, the legions of people who had passed through his centers. He knew, because he had gone through it himself. He, like so many others, had been written off, told by his doctors to watch his diet, don't exercise, take a nap after lunch.

Thus, in one aspect, the power of Nathan Pritikin's message is in voices like those in this book. People who listened and understood, because they had no alternative. The acutely ill, who had run out of options. Individuals like Alan Keiser. What concern did he have for neat pages of scientifically valid figures? Conventional medicine had run out of options for him.

Modern medicine has been criticized for not being sensitive enough to the difference between medicine and health. Aided by its powerful ally, technology, medical science has become extremely skilled at saving lives. Without the heart-lung machine, without the computerized monitoring of the ICU and sensitive surgical instrumentation, bypass surgery would be impossible. Remember that before bypass, a high percentage of men with heart disease were dead four years after its onset. Without technology, the complicated life-saving diagnostic technique of angiography would never have been developed. Medicine has become big business, representing some ten percent of our gross national product. That's wonderful for employment, but not much so when you realize that all this technology is not equally available to everyone. More importantly, and this is the thrust of Nathan's message, it doesn't need to be. The old adage is true: an ounce of prevention is worth a pound of cure.

Although many health professionals were interested in the Pritikin Program because of its potential to aid the critically ill, many others were attracted by its possibilities for prevention. Nathan professed not to recognize the difference. He wanted everybody on his diet. He stuck strictly to his numbers and refused to consider compromise. His critics, and even sometimes his colleagues, might suggest that it would be better for more people to be on a modified Pritikin Program instead of fewer people on it in its purest form. Nathan wasn't interested.

In effect Nathan Pritikin had a powerful tool for people in whom heredity and life-style had conspired to produce atherosclerosis and heart disease. It appeared from my sample that few researchers working in this area would dispute that premise: drastic measures for a difficult disease. What he also had, and here he was less successful in implementation, was the core of a prevention program—a program that, with the right kind of education, could prevent large numbers of people from developing heart disease, even despite, as we saw in Martin Stone's case, unfavorable heredity. Dr. William Castelli once suggested to me that he suspected most American households had about ten sample meals that were routinely rotated, and if you could just plug into that pattern, you'd have it made. What if those ten meals were loaded with complex carbohydrates and chicken and vegetables instead of steak and lemon chiffon pie?

Nathan Pritikin was overly optimistic in his predictions that half of the population of this country would be adhering to the Pritikin diet by 1985. But the real message in his words is that if we played our cards right, we wouldn't have to. If we started off on the right track from the beginning, we wouldn't have to resort to such drastic measures to regain our health. Perhaps Nathan should have settled for a fifty percent awareness of where our fast-paced, high-stress life-style is taking us, full as we are of greasy hamburgers and French-fried potatoes, or rich ice cream and heavy sauces and empty snacks. We have taken steps, that is sure, and research and medicine will continue to assess various approaches to "teaching" people about diet. Dr. Robert Levy's NIH study clearly linked high cholesterol with heart disease. Framingham continues to refine its determination of heart disease risk factors.

Although he himself may not have reached as many people as he would have liked, Nathan Pritikin set the wheels in motion. By being inflexible, by refusing to deviate, by making his unilateral statements, he forced people to listen. And listen they did. Our social institutions change slowly; that, in fact, is one of their functions, in order to protect society from harmful fads and ill-founded suppositions. But, given adequate pressure from society or its leaders, institutions do move forward. And Nathan Pritikin had the capacity to inspire the type of social movement that presses toward that kind of constructive change.

Nathan's legacy cannot be calculated solely in the numbers of people, sick or well, that adhere to his program, but rather in the number of people who are aware that a diet rich in fat, cholesterol and refined carbohydrates is bad for your health. It can be found in the salad bars that have suddenly sprung up in the fast-food hamburger joints, in the expanded fish sections of steak-house menus, in the nonfat dairy products that can be more easily found on supermarket shelves. When I first started my work with Nathan, I had to make my own nonfat yogurt. Now I can buy it in my supermarket dairy section. Nathan's legacy is there, in the decline of red meat sales, in the admission of the national beef lobby that Americans now "prefer smaller amounts of red meat." It can be detected in every conversation with the person who tells you he or she only eats fish or chicken now, swearing off the steaks and chops. Perhaps no image is more telling than that of food aficionados Craig Claiborne and the late James Beard admitting their doctors' recommendations for reducing the amount of salt in their diets.

Although it didn't happen fast enough to satisfy him, Nathan's legacy lies in our increasing national awareness that the type of food we eat is related to health—that the "three squares" and the four food groups aren't all we have to know about food to keep us healthy. And that a sedentary life-style is deadly.

When I first learned of Nathan's death, my initial reaction was that he didn't accomplish all that he wanted to, that he didn't get everything done. The thought produced a sadness, then an enlightenment: Nathan's legacy is that he raised our consciousness. As hackneyed as that phrase has come to be, the reality is that he did get us to think. He may not have had all the answers—a nation's health, after all, is a complicated matter—but he helped start it all, against all odds. Let us hope that in the future we can reduce the arbitrary choice between the "typical American diet" and the strict routine that Nathan advocated. Let us hope that we can adopt moderation in all our habits, from the time we are born, and learn the need to make choices. Let us hope, as was Nathan's dream, that the "typical American diet" will be a low-fat, low-cholesterol diet.

Speaking of his brother at the time of his death, Albert Pritikin remarked that Nathan belonged to everyone and yet was close to no one. There's no doubt that, given the deepest recesses of his thoughts and desires, Nathan Pritikin was a very private man. He was introspective, but at the same time he was accessible and vocal to the many people who sought him out, as we have seen in these pages. Ironically, he was a loner who influenced the lives of thousands of people and the thoughts of millions more.

Let's hope he knew it.

Glossary of Terms

Aneurysm—the ballooning-out of the wall of a vein or artery or the heart, usually due to disease or injury, although it may be abnormally present at birth.

Angina pectoris—pain in the front and middle of the chest, tending to radiate down either arm or up the neck to the jaw. The pain is usually attributed to a temporary scarcity of blood to one or more areas of the heart.

Artery—a blood vessel that carries blood from the heart to the various parts of the body.

Angiogram—an X ray of the arteries of the heart, taken by injecting radiopaque material separately into the right and left coronary artery after which a series of X rays are rapidly taken.

Atherosclerosis—a condition in which the inner layers of an artery wall are thickened by deposits composed chiefly of cholesterol and fat.

Atrium—one of the two upper chambers of the heart.

Blood pressure—the force, or pressure, exerted by the heart as it pumps blood; also refers to the pressure of blood as it flows through the arteries.

CAPD—continuous ambulatory peritoneal dialysis—a method of dialysis that uses the peritoneal lining of the abdomen to simulate the action of the kidneys.

Cardiac—of or pertaining to the heart.

Cardiac arrest—condition occurring when the heart stops beating, which effectively means the cessation of blood flow and effective circulation.

Cardiovascular—relating to the heart and blood vessels.

Cholesterol—a fat-like, pearly substance found in all animal fat and oils, in bile, blood, and brain tissue; cholesterol is necessary to produce certain hormones and construct cells.

Collateral circulation—the development of a system of smaller blood vessels that carry blood when a main vessel is blocked.

Coronary arteries—two arteries that rise out of the aorta (the main trunk artery that receives blood from the lower left chamber of the heart) down over the top of the heart, carrying blood to the heart muscle.

Coronary—a heart attack; also known by the medical term myocardial infarction.

Coronary artery disease—a generally symptomless disorder in which one or more of the coronary arteries is partially or totally obstructed.

Coronary thrombosis—clot in a coronary artery obstructing blood flow.

Diabetes—a chronic disorder in the body's ability to metabolize carbohydrates, resulting from a disturbance in normal insulin function.

Digitalis—a drug strengthening the contractions of the heart and promoting elimination of fluids from the body.

Diuretic—a substance promoting the excretion of urine.

Fibrillation—uncoordinated contractions occurring when individual muscle fibers in the heart contract irregularly.

Hemodialysis (hemo)—conventional method of dialysis, in which the patient's blood is filtered through a kidney dialysis machine.

Hypercholesteremia—excess cholesterol in the blood.

Hypertension—an unstable or persistent elevation of blood pressure above normal.

Ischemic heart disease—coronary heart disease.

Lipoprotein—combination of a lipid (fat) with protein molecules in the blood. (Lipids don't dissolve in the blood and are thus carried in this configuration.)

Low density lipoprotein—those that carry most of the cholesterol circulating in the blood. An elevated LDL level is a major risk factor for heart disease.

High density lipoprotein—although a carrier of cholesterol, HDLs are considered to transport cholesterol from the tissues to the liver so that it can be excreted in the bile.

Myocardial infarction—damage or death of an area of heart muscle from a reduction in blood supply to that area.

Nitroglycerin—drug causing dilation of the blood vessels.

Plaque—a scar-like mass in an artery that contains varying amounts of cholesterol, fat and possibly calcium.

Stress—physical or mental tension that can be caused by physical, chemical or emotional factors. The term can also refer to physical exertion as well as mental anxiety.

Vein—one of a series of blood vessels carrying blood from various parts of the body back to the heart.

Ventricle—one of the two lower chambers of the heart.

About the Author

Penelope Grenoble has had fifteen years of experience in the fields of communications and health, including work with such organizations as the U. S. Public Health Service, the Veterans Administration and the Departments of Health and Human Services, as well as being a former editor-in-chief of the *Los Angeles Free Press*. As executive director of the Pritikin Research Foundation her responsibilities included the routine interviewing of Pritikin Longevity Center alumni for program updates. Dr. Grenoble holds a Ph.D. in Communication and Rhetoric from Rensselaer Polytechnic Institute, is the author, with Robert Soll, M.D., Ph.D., of *MS — Something Can Be Done and You Can Do It,* and has written extensively on a variety of subjects for newspapers, magazines, journals, and film and video production. She lives with her husband in California.